OPHTHALMOLOGIC NURSING

OPHTHALMOLOGIC NURSING

JOAN F. SMITH, Ph.D, R.N.
Assistant Professor of Nursing,
Medical Surgical Nursing Department,
The University of Michigan School of Nursing,
Ann Arbor

DELBERT P. NACHAZEL, JR., M.D.
Assistant Clinical Professor of Ophthalmology,
Wayne State University School of Medicine,
Detroit

Attending Surgeon,
William Beaumont Hospital,
Royal Oak, Michigan

Little, Brown and Company, Boston

Library of Congress Catalog Card No. 79-92960

ISBN 0-316-80158-5

Printed in the United States of America

HAL

Photography by:

Frank Flanagin,
Associated Retinal Consultants of Detroit, Michigan (Drs. Nachazel, Margherio, Murphy and Cox)

Czaba L. Martonyi,
Department of Ophthalmology,
The University of Michigan

Artist:

Hedwig Murphy

PREFACE

Ophthalmologic Nursing is intended for undergraduate and graduate students of nursing and for nurses who need ready access to specialized eye care information. It will be most helpful to nurses who work in primary care settings, occupational health settings, or extended practice, and to those who work in secondary care settings, emergency rooms, extended care facilities, tertiary care settings, acute care settings, or chronic long-term care settings.

The book has been organized according to an anatomic format, which allows the reader to analyze logically the problem at hand. This organization is useful for the nurse because it parallels techniques of patient assessment by looking first at the eye's outermost structure. Therefore the first chapter discusses the eyelids, conjunctiva, and lacrimal system. The common ophthalmologic problems are dealt with, as are those seen less frequently.

The nurse clinician will find information to help her assess the patient's condition and plan rehabilitative care. The nursing care discussions include the sociological and psychological aspects of care for ophthalmologic patients. The cognitive knowledge related to emergency care applies the cardinal rule to evaluate gross vision before "laying on hands."

The book has two sections. Part I covers the anatomy, histology, and pathophysiology needed as background for nursing assessment, intervention, and treatment. Special diagnostic tests and instruments used for eye examination are also discussed.

Part II consists of three chapters. One of these chapters describes the physical assessment of the eye. Primary assessment skills are being taught to nurses in undergraduate and graduate nursing programs and are used by nurse clinicians in various health-care settings. The techniques for physical assessment and the most commonly used instruments are described. A chapter on the most commonly used nursing measures deals with techniques as varied as instilling eyedrops and cleaning a prosthesis. A chapter on blindness provides some helpful hints for the rehabilitation of the visually disabled person. It also informs the nurse of ways to provide a safe hospital, home, and community environment for the visually disabled patient.

The scope of ophthalmologic nursing is expanding. Nurses are increasingly active as health-care providers, and their need for information has also increased. *Ophthalmologic Nursing* is designed to meet these needs.

We would like to express our gratitude to those who have assisted us in reading this manuscript. We are especially appreciative and grateful to Dr. John W. Henderson, Professor of Ophthalmology and past chairperson of Ophthalmology at The University of Michigan, for reading the entire manuscript and making helpful suggestions. Our thanks to Mary Lou Frey, Assistant Professor of Nursing at The University of Michigan School of Nursing; Evelyn Johnson, staff nurse at General Motors Technical Center; Victor Irving of Blind Services; and Cam Williams of the Occupational Therapy Department, The Rehabilitation Institute of Detroit. Our thanks also to Julie Stillman, Nursing Department Editor, and Helane Manditch-Prottas, Copyediting Supervisor, of Little, Brown and Company and other members of the staff for their support during the writing and publishing of this book.

J. F. S.
D. P. N.

CONTENTS

NOTICE

The indications and dosages of all drugs in this book have been recommended in the medical literature and conform to the practices of the general medical community. The medications described do not necessarily have specific approval by the Food and Drug Administration for use in the diseases and dosages for which they are recommended. The package insert for each drug should be consulted for use and dosage as approved by the FDA. Because standards for usage change, it is advisable to keep abreast of revised recommendations, particularly those concerning new drugs.

PART I ———————————

ANATOMY, HISTOLOGY, PHYSIOLOGY, PATHOLOGY: MEDICAL TREATMENT AND NURSING CARE

CHAPTER 1

EYELIDS, CONJUNCTIVA, AND LACRIMAL SYSTEM

ANATOMY

EYELID

The *eyelid* is divided into several distinct layers. The skin is some of the thinnest in the body. The subcutaneous layer of the lid consists of loose connective tissue; the muscle layer has fibers in a roughly horizontal alignment (Fig. 1–1). The muscle of the lid, called the *orbicularis oculi,* is supplied by the seventh cranial (facial) nerve and functions to close the lid. The submuscular connective tissue contains the nerves to the eyelid. The tarsal plate, a dense mass of fibrous tissue, gives shape and firmness to each lid. There is no cartilage present in these plates. The meibomian glands are incorporated within the tarsal plate and exit on the margin of the lid just in front of its posterior border. There are about 20 to 25 glands in each lid. These are modified sebaceous glands that produce an oily secretion to prevent (1) overflow of tears and (2) maceration of the skin of the lid by the tears. The *levator palpebrae* muscle inserts on the anterior surface of the superior tarsal plate. It is innervated by the third cranial (oculomotor) nerve and functions to elevate the upper lid. The small gray line just anterior to the orifices of the meibomian glands marks the potential space between the orbicularis muscle and the tarsal plate, delineating the anterior and posterior sections of the lid. The lid may be separated easily by incising through the gray line. This anatomic division is important in many plastic surgical procedures of the lid. There is a very thin layer of vertically aligned muscle fiber just behind the tarsus, and this layer and the conjunctiva are tightly adherent to the tarsus.

The lashes exit from the skin of the lid anterior to the gray line. Attached to each lash follicle are the *glands of Zeis.* There are usually two or more glands to each lash follicle. When infected, these glands become swollen and are called *hordeolum* or *stye.* Another type, *Moll's glands,* arrested sweat gland, are in the skin

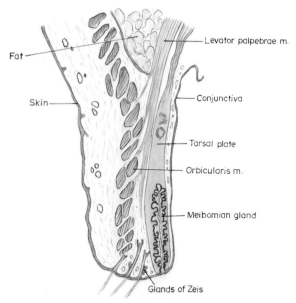

Figure 1–1. *Cross section of lid.*

near the lid margin. When infected, they also are called *hordeolum* or *stye.*

CONJUNCTIVA

The *conjunctiva* is a thin transparent mucous membrane that forms a continuous covering of the inner surface of the lid and then is reflected onto the anterior portion of the eyeball, eventually becoming continuous with the epithelium of the cornea (Fig. 1–2). The conjunctiva is divided roughly into three sections: the palpebral, covering the inner lid; the bulbar, covering the globe; and the area between the two, the fornix. The palpebral conjunctiva is tightly adherent to the tarsus and it is difficult to dissect them. The bulbar conjunctiva and the fornix have looser attachments and are easily movable across the underlying structures.

LACRIMAL SYSTEM

The *lacrimal system* consists of several major components: the lacrimal gland, the punctum, the canaliculus, the lacrimal sac, and the nasolacrimal duct (Fig. 1–3). The lacrimal gland lies in the

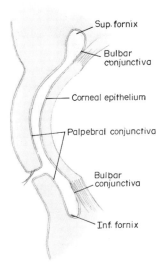

Figure 1–2. *Cross section of conjunctiva and adjacent structures.*

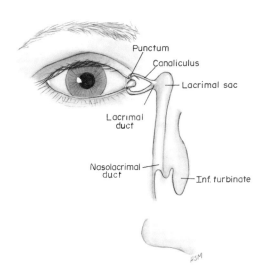

Figure 1–3. *Lacrimal duct system.*

upper temporal portion of the orbit, it is about 20 mm by 12 mm in size. The largest portion of the gland lies in apposition to the inner bony wall of the orbit just above the upper lid. It is held in place by attachments in the periosteum in this area. Its anterior third lies behind the temporal part of the upper lid. The gland is very soft in consistency and cannot be palpated unless it becomes swollen. The ducts exit from the anterior portion of the gland into the superior temporal conjunctival fornix.

The tears flow across the eye and are moved nasally along the superior margin of the lower lid to the lower punctum. Some flow occurs through the upper punctum, but most occurs through the lower. The punctum is the entrance into the tear duct system. This consists of a small opening several millimeters temporal to the nasal edge of the upper and lower lid. The punctum opens into a narrow channel called a *lacrimal canaliculus,* which runs horizontally along the upper portion of the remainder of the nasal part of the upper and lower lid margin and then usually joins with its fellow, forming a common lacrimal duct that enters into the lacrimal sac. The lacrimal sac is about 15 mm long and 5 mm in diameter. It is the upper dilated portion of the nasolacrimal duct and it lies in the lacrimal fossa, a slight depression just behind the inferior orbital rim, where the rim meets the base of the nose. The nasolacrimal canal is a bony canal that extends into the nose from the lacrimal fossa. Its mucosal lining is the nasolacrimal duct, which carries excess tears into the nose. Thus, weeping may cause the excess tears to flow into the nose, resulting in a watery nasal discharge.

DISORDERS OF THE LIDS

INFECTIONS

Hordeolum and Chalazion

The term *stye* commonly designates an infected swelling near the lid margin. There are two types: internal and external. An internal stye is an infection of the meibomian gland and is called a *chalazion* (Figs. 1-4, 1-5). An external stye is an infection of the glands of Moll or Zeis and is called a *hordeolum.* Either of these infections may cause a marked swollen and reddened lid. Usually an acute stye will involve only one lid at a time, but there may be evidence of an incipient infection in the other lid. Closer inspec-

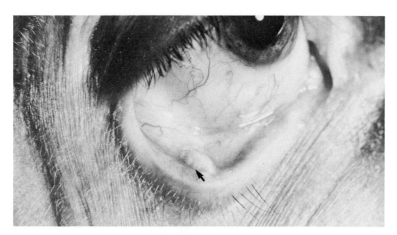

Figure 1-4. *Chalazion (arrow). Appearance of conjunctival surface. (Photo courtesy of Csaba L. Martonyi, Department of Ophthalmology, The University of Michigan Medical School.)*

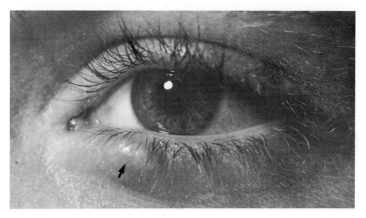

Figure 1-5. *Chalazion (arrow). External appearance of lid. (Photo courtesy of Csaba L. Martonyi, Department of Ophthalmology, The University of Michigan Medical School.)*

tion will demonstrate either swelling or pointing of one of the ducts along the lash line (hordeolum) or pointing along the mouth of a meibomian gland (chalazion).

If there is difficulty in making the diagnosis, the lid can be everted and, in the case of a chalazion, inflammation in the tarsus will show through the tarsal conjunctiva. If the lid is so swollen that a differential diagnosis cannot be made, a standard treatment of compresses and antibiotic eyedrops or ointments should be initiated. Usually the lid edema resolves and a definitive diagnosis can be made. Treatment may then need to be adjusted.

Hordeolum are of short duration often resolving within several days. As the lesion forms, filling with pus, there is a sharp pain that becomes dull and throbbing. When the lesion is opened (either by warm compresses and spontaneous rupture or by incision) pus escapes and the pain ceases.

Warm compresses applied four times a day are helpful not only to bring the hordeolum to a head and allow an adequate rupture and drainage of its infected contents, but to relieve the discomfort. This pyogenic infection can be incised, if it does not evacuate spontaneously, but should never be squeezed, since infected material may be expressed into the venous system of the face and eyelids and be transmitted to the brain through the superior ophthalmic vein or the inferior ophthalmic vein or both.

An antibiotic (neomycin or chloramphenicol) may be used at bedtime. While antibiotics are used, they are not necessary, as styes are generally gone within a few days (treated or untreated). Some feel that the antibiotic is helpful to prevent infection to the subsequent neighboring glands at the base of the lash.

Chalazions, on the other hand, are more chronic and will often quiet but not completely resorb. They remain as a cystlike swelling in the lid and usually reactivate within months. If reactivation occurs, a large cyst will remain, and excision of the cyst is the best method of treatment. Excision is performed by infiltrating the lid with a local anesthetic, clamping and everting the lid with a special chalazion lid clamp, and incising into the cyst through the tarsal conjunctiva. A small curette is then used to scrape out the caseous material that is always found in these chronic chalazions. Most surgeons also attempt to excise some or all of the wall of the cyst.

When the infection is acute, this cystic formation can cause pressure on the cornea and some discomfort, especially when the upper lid is closed. Discomfort is more pronounced if a secondary infection develops and purulent material accumulates. Massaging the lid margin may be helpful to maintain normal flow and prevent the other glands from becoming infected. An antibiotic or sulfonamide eyedrop often is used three or four times a day before and after surgery. Sulfacetamide sodium (Sodium Sulamyd) or a combination drug like Neosporin is usually satisfactory.

Chalazions often cause sensitivity to light. Epiphora (persistent weeping) may occur. Meibomitis is usually associated with a chalazion and may contribute to the sensation of tired eyes. Because of this weeping and tired eyes, ointments are soothing and may be useful at night.

Blepharitis

Blepharitis is a chronic infection of the glands and lash follicles along the lid margin (Fig. 1–6). The most common causes are staphylococcal and seborrheic. Staphylococcal infections are associated with hard, tenacious scales that are frequently difficult to remove. There are occasional ulcers along the lid margin, and acne or other skin infections such as styes are often present.

The seborrheic type shows greasy, easily removed scales, is always bilateral, and is associated with seborrheic dermatitis of the scalp and often of brows and external ears. Conjunctivitis is usually not present as may be the case with staphylococcal blepharitis. Common symptoms found in patients with blepharitis are pruritus, pain, light sensitivity, epiphora, and "tired eyes." The patient's general health should be evaluated. The cause of the problem may be a focal infection in the mouth or nasopharynx. The patient may have any of the following: anemia, gout, diabetes, or allergy. At times, uncleanliness and poor diet contribute to blepharitis. A well-balanced diet is essential, with additional fruits and fruit juices giving more vitamins A, B, and D.

A definitive diagnosis can be made by microscopic examination of the lid scrapings. However, it is common to have a mixed infection of scalp and eyelids. In such cases, the seborrheic component of the scalp should be treated first with an antifungal shampoo (Selsun or Sebulex).

In blepharitis the eyelids may become glued shut with mucus type discharge. This dries and crusts on the lids. Scaling of the skin under this mucous crusty discharge becomes a problem. The scaling, exudates, and crusts can be removed with warm compresses, which will soften the dried secretions. Olive oil or hydrogen peroxide can be used to soften and free the crusts from the lashes. The oil or hydrogen peroxide can be applied to the eyelids with cotton pledgets, stroking downward and sideways to remove the thick mucinous exudate. An appropriate antibiotic eyedrop three or four times a day should be used to treat the infective component of the blepharitis. If skin infection is present, systemic or topical antibiotics may be necessary.

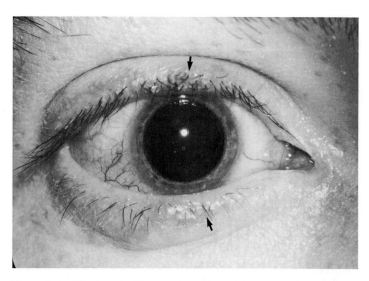

Figure 1–6. *Blepharitis. Note scaling along lid margins (arrows). (Photo courtesy of Sally A. Rourke, Department of Ophthalmology, The University of Michigan Medical School.)*

Meibomitis

Meibomitis is an infection of the meibomian glands. It is different from a chalazion in that the ducts are not occluded and a cyst does not form. In its acute form, meibomitis is usually accompanied by chalazion or blepharitis. In its chronic form, mild irritation and burning may accompany meibomitis. It can be diagnosed by exerting minimal pressure just above the lid margin while watching the orifices of the meibomian glands under a slit lamp. The secretions that are expressed will be cloudy rather than the amber, clear fluid that is normally present.

Treatment consists of warm compresses, two to four times a day, applied with a clean washcloth each time or sterile 4 by 4 in. gauze squares. The patient may sit at the sink with warm running water and apply compresses for approximately 3 to 4 minutes. The washcloth can be refolded, always with a clean portion toward the affected eye. Because the ducts are occluded, tarsal massage twice a day is helpful in clearing the ducts. Massage should be performed at the lid margin immediately following the application of compresses. The person who is massaging may see the cloudy secretions disappear and the normal clear amber fluid being expressed. An appropriate antibiotic eyedrop or ointment may be used. As the day goes on, the eyes may become tired and irritated. An ointment applied to the lid margins at bedtime is therefore quite soothing.

ABNORMALITIES OF THE LID POSITION

Entropion

Entropion is a condition caused by inversion of the lid resulting in the lid margin and lashes rubbing on the eyeball. There are two types: (1) cicatricial, caused by distortion in the conjunctiva or tarsus and (2) spastic, caused by contraction of the orbicularis muscle near the lid margin. Cicatricial entropion usually involves the upper lid. The cause is usually trauma or a burn. Spastic, the more common variety, usually involves the lower lid, and often occurs in the elderly who are predisposed to it because of laxness of the lid supporting tissue. Symptoms result from corneal irritation and may include pain, tearing, conjunctival infection, and corneal ulceration.

Initial treatment for spastic entropion involves splinting the lid, which may be done by using a pressure patch or by taping the lid into its normal position. If a patch is applied, the lid must be in its normal position before the patch is applied, and the patch must be applied firmly enough to prevent the lid from rolling after application. Occasionally, patching or splinting may relieve eye irritation and break the cycle of irritation, spasm, more irritation, worse spasm. Usually, surgery is necessary for spastic entropion and is always necessary for cicatricial entropion.

Many surgical procedures have been developed, and they are based on one of two basic approaches. One, the orbicularis procedure, is to tighten the musculature along the edge of the tarsus farthest away from the lid margin, thus everting the lid margin (Fig. 1–7). The other is to remove a triangle from the tarsal plate with its base at the edge of the tarsal plate farthest away from the lid margin (Fig. 1–8). Then, by suturing the defect made during the procedure, the peripheral part of the tarsus is tightened and the lid margin is approximated to the eyeball. This latter technique is the basis for most of the procedures and it works well.

Postoperatively, the eye is patched. The care of the patient then is the same as for any monocular sighted individual. (See Chap. 8, Partially Sighted Patients.) The patient may receive an antibiotic type eyedrop several times a day to prevent infection.

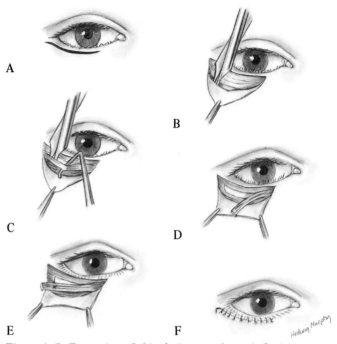

Figure 1–7. *Entropion. Orbicularis procedure. A. Incision along lid margin. B. Exposure of orbicularis muscle. C. and D. Dislocation of an inferior band of orbicularis fibers. E. Shortened inferior orbicularis muscle band. F. Skin closure.*

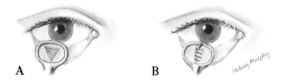

Figure 1–8. *Entropion. Tarsal resection.*

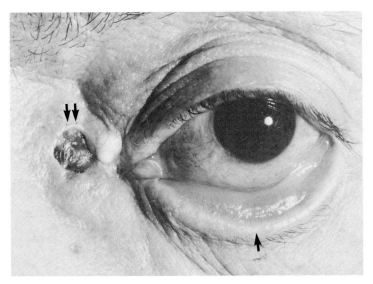

Figure 1-9. *Ectropion (single arrow). Nonrelated sebaceous cyst (double arrow). (Photo courtesy of Csaba L. Martonyi, Department of Ophthalmology, The University of Michigan Medical School.)*

Ectropion

Ectropion is the condition caused by eversion of the lid margin (Fig. 1-9). There are multiple causes: (1) senile, from laxness of the skin and orbicularis muscle, always involving the lower lid, (2) paralytic, also involving the lower lid is caused by a facial nerve paralysis, (3) mechanical, caused by edema of the palpebral conjunctiva, and (4) cicatricial, caused by contraction of scar tissue.

Spastic ectropion frequently can be treated successfully by patching. If the paralysis becomes permanent, surgical correction is necessary. Surgery is always necessary in cicatricial and advanced senile ectropion.

The results of ectropion surgery are rather predictable. A full-thickness base-up triangle of skin, tarsus, and conjunctiva is removed with the base of the triangle at the lid margin. The defect is then closed in a linear vertical fashion, usually in three layers (Fig. 1-10). The lid margin must be level at the end of the procedure; otherwise, a notch will form at the lid margin as healing occurs. Antibiotic ointment is used prophylactically.

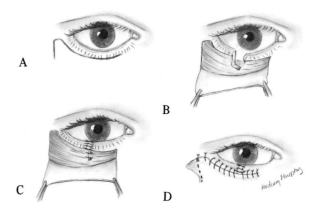

Figure 1–10. *Ectropion repair. A. Skin incision. B. Excision of wedge of conjunctiva, tarsus, and muscle. C. Closure of wedge resection. D. Closure of skin with removal of excess tissue temporally.*

Patching after the first day or two depends on patient comfort.

Nursing care revolves around presurgical and postsurgical treatment. Occasionally, control of conjunctival infection and irritation may prevent the need for surgery in early senile or mechanical ectropion. Topical antibiotics along with patching and compresses are indicated. Postoperatively, care should follow the same guidelines as postoperative entropion surgery.

Ptosis

Ptosis means a lowering of the upper lid so that it partly or completely covers the cornea. It is usually associated with weakness in the levator superioris muscle (Fig. 1–11). Ptosis usually occurs as a congenital defect but it can be associated with damage secondary to trauma. It is often the first sign of myasthenia gravis. Paralysis, usually partial, of the levator superioris is the underlying pathology.

Two basic types of operations are used depending on the severity of the levator superioris muscle paralysis. If the paralysis is very great, a sling is fashioned to hold the lid in an acceptable position. This operation is performed by inserting a band or suture under the skin in a manner that will support the lid. The foreign material is threaded along the margin of the upper lid and then vertically to a position above the brow where it is tied as tightly as neces-

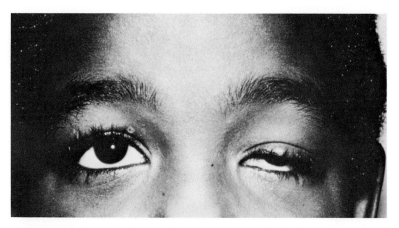

Figure 1-11. *Ptosis, left eye. (Photo courtesy of Csaba L. Martonyi, Department of Ophthalmology, The University of Michigan Medical School.)*

sary to raise the lid to the desired level. The entire foreign material is buried under the skin. If the muscle paralysis is not too great, the muscle can be shortened to increase its power. This is done by isolating the levator palpebrae superioris muscle, severing its attachment to the superior edge of the tarsus, and reattaching the muscle to the tarsus at a level higher on the muscle. This shortens the muscle and gives added strength. Either of these operations is effective, depending on the individual's condition. The sling operation gives a reasonably good cosmetic result but does not improve function. The muscle shortening operation often restores good function.

Ptosis can be unilateral or bilateral. It can be slight or it can be severe enough that the pupil is covered by the upper lid. This of course causes vision to be obstructed and is also annoying.

Patients use compensatory mechanisms to try to overcome the pupillary obstruction. They raise or elevate the eyebrow or contract the frontalis muscle and tilt their head back. These measures are annoying and frequently lead one to seek medical attention.

Surgery can be performed to correct this drooping lid. If for some reason surgery is contraindicated, glasses with a crutch can be worn. The small crutch elevates the drooping eyelid.

PREOPERATIVE NURSING CARE. Patients are admitted the day before surgery and have the routine laboratory work done. If patients are over 40 years of age, and some of these patients are, an ECG is run. However, the majority of patients seen with ptosis are children or young adults.

The evening before surgery the patient receives a sedative to allow him a good night's sleep. Generally the patients take nothing by mouth from midnight the evening before surgery.

The morning of surgery, the patient receives a preoperative medication of a narcotic such as meperidine (Demerol) and a narcotic potentiator or tranquilizer such as promethazine hydrochloride (Phenergan) or hydroxyzine pamoate (Vistaril) intramuscularly. Since general anesthesia is usually used the patient also receives atropine intramuscularly to aid in eliminating secretions and to make the induction phase of anesthesia less difficult. At this time, the patient frequently receives an antibiotic or sulfa type eyedrop to lower the pathogens in the conjunctiva. These medications are usually given one hour preoperatively. An oral sedative may be given 1½ hours preoperatively; frequently it is the same medication given the evening before surgery.

POSTOPERATIVE NURSING CARE. The patient is returned to the room, and the nursing care is similar to that for any surgical patient. Vital signs should be taken until they are stable.

The patient is permitted out of bed to the bathroom with assistance when the effects of the anesthetic are gone. Since the surgery involves the lid, and is not intraocular, any comfortable position may be maintained. Patient's diet is returned to the regular full diet as soon as it is tolerated.

Generally patients do not complain of pain, but there is a slight headache or discomfort in the lid region. Tylenol, one or two tablets, No. 3 (Tylenol gr V with ½ gr of codeine) or Tylenol gr X generally suffices. If nausea and vomiting occur, an antiemetic is ordered whenever necessary.

The eye is patched before return from the operating room to keep the area clean and to protect the eye from the irritation of artificial light or sunlight. There may be some swelling or edema of the eyelid. Generally, upon changing the eyepatch, one notes a moderate amount of serosanguineous type discharge. Often the eyelid is sutured closed for the first 24 hours to avoid exposure of the cornea beneath the dressing.

Sometimes there is overcorrection in ptosis surgery, although this is rare. If overcorrection occurs, an antibiotic ointment is applied to the eye to protect the cornea until the lid adjusts, or further surgery is done to resolve the overcorrection. If further surgery is necessary, the lid is separated and the tarsus is stretched in hopes of spreading the lid sufficiently so that the lid closes and the cornea is not exposed. An antibiotic or steroid type drop is usually instilled four times a day for prophylactic prevention of drying or infection of the cornea.

Patients generally are discharged in several days and return to the doctor's office in a week for removal of sutures. Patients continue to instill the steroid or antibiotic eyedrop four times a day until they are seen at the doctor's office.

Blepharochalasis

Blepharochalasis is excessive lid tissue due to atrophy and relaxation of tissue of the upper lids (Fig. 1–12). In some instances the loose skin may fold over the margin of the lid and mechanically obstruct vision. Surgery is necessary to correct the problem. Treatment is excision of the excess skin. The cosmetic and functional results are usually very good.

Nursing care is minimal, as these patients may have surgery on an outpatient basis. The eye is patched to prevent irritation from the light as well as to keep the operative site clean. Discomfort is minimal, and a mild analgesic may be given if necessary.

TUMORS

Nonmalignant Tumors

There are many types of nonmalignant tumors of the lid. Most, however, are benign papillomas and are not in themselves of concern. The primary diagnostic concern is to ascertain whether a malignant tumor is mimicking a nonmalignant tumor. Consequently, the physician must maintain a high index of suspicion. A questionable lesion should be biopsied, and even relatively large lesions can be removed in toto without disfigurement. Because of the looseness of the skin of the lid, lidplasty can easily be performed to cover defects caused by such biopsies.

One particularly obvious type of nonmalignant tumor is the xanthelasma—yellowish, elevated lesion that almost invariably begins on the nasal side of the upper or lower lid (Fig. 1–13). It may extend in a relatively narrow ribbon temporally the full length of the lid. It is common to see xanthelasma on all four lids. There are no symptoms, and hence no treatment is required unless the patient desires cosmetic improvement. Most ophthalmol-

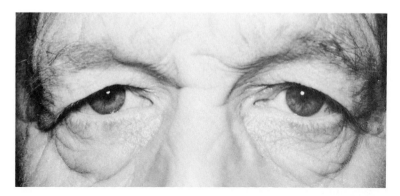

Figure 1-12. *Blepharochalasis, upper lid. (Photo courtesy of Frank Flanagin, Associated Retinal Consultants, Detroit.)*

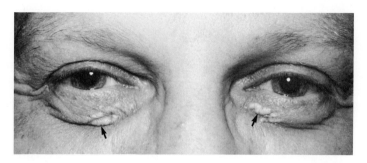

Figure 1-13. *Xanthelasma. Arrows point to placques. (Photo courtesy of Csaba L. Martonyi, Department of Ophthalmology, The University of Michigan Medical School.)*

ogists prefer to surgically excise these lesions. However, acid therapy or electrodiathermy may be used. Cosmetic results are usually good no matter what method is used. It is well to note that there is a relationship between xanthelasma and blood cholesterol and fat levels in some patients.

Malignant Tumors

BASAL CELL CARCINOMA. Basal cell carcinoma is the most common malignant tumor of the lid. It is usually seen on the lower lid and has the appearance of a firm mound of smooth tissue. It may or may not have an ulceration in its center. If unattended, these tumors enlarge to a remarkable size. However, they are slow growing and can be treated effectively with radiation therapy or surgical removal.

SQUAMOUS CELL CARCINOMAS. Squamous cell carcinomas are more often seen on the upper lid, are more invasive, show more ulceration and, as a general rule, are much more rapidly growing than basal cell carcinoma. Squamous cell carcinomas are much more radio resistant, but are also not so amenable to surgical removal as are basal cell carcinomas. It is extremely important that these be recognized and treated early. Often, the only way to make a sound diagnosis is to biopsy the lesion, since the appearance may not be characteristic.

INJURIES

Lacerations

Lacerations can be caused by either a sharp or blunt blow. If a laceration does occur, one must be concerned about the integrity of the globe beneath the lid. The eyeball itself is the first consideration in an injury severe enough to cause a lid laceration. Lacerations of the lid can extend to the cornea and conjunctiva, and the globe of the eye should be examined for any such occurrence (Fig. 1–14). Before beginning to care for any injured person, vision should be evaluated. A gross examination, such as count fingers or "read the top line of the Snellen's chart," is sufficient. From a medical standpoint (to plan treatment), and from a medicolegal standpoint, it is important to have some kind of vision screening done before examination or treatment is initiated.

Treatment in most instances involves primary repair of the laceration. The nurse washes the lids gently with saline and surgical soap. The surgeon then anesthetizes the area and prepares to suture the edges of the lids together. Depending on the severity of the injury, this can be a relatively simple operation or a very time-consuming and difficult plastic repair. Most simple lacerations can be closed with the patient under local anesthetic, and, if the edges are sharp, the laceration can be sutured directly edge-to-edge. It is extremely important that exact apposition occur at the lash line; if the laceration should carry through the eyebrow, it is also important that this repair be approximated meticulously. Both the anterior and posterior portion of the laceration should be sutured

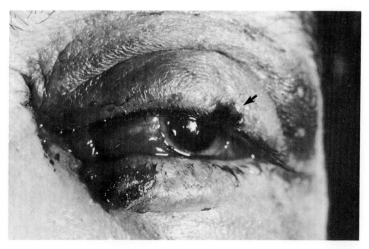

Figure 1–14. *Lid laceration. A notch in upper lid tissue to be excised. (Photo courtesy of Csaba L. Martonyi, Department of Ophthalmology, The University of Michigan Medical School.)*

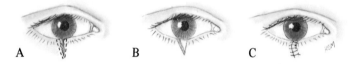

Figure 1–15. *Repair of lid laceration. A. Dotted lines show lacerated tissue to be excised. B. Freshened wound. C. Primary repair completed.*

if it is a through-and-through laceration. Most surgeons would prefer to see a laceration closed so that there is a slight mound on the lid margin at the site of closure. The tissue does tend to shrink slightly when it scars, and a small notching may occur at the lid margin if this technique is not observed. Certainly if the laceration is not a clean one, this technique of developing a slight mound at the wound margin is more important (Fig. 1–15). If the laceration is quite jagged, the macerated tissue should be excised before closure is attempted.

A complication of a lid laceration occurs when the laceration extends through one or both of the canaliculi at the nasal margin of the lid. This is most unfortunate if the lower canaliculus is involved, since the lower canaliculus carries most of the tear flow

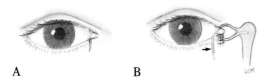

A   B

Figure 1-16. *Canaliculus repair. Stent (arrow)*
has been threaded through canaliculus. A.
Laceration through canaliculus. B. Laceration
closed with a stent through canaliculus.

into the lacrimal sac. It is extremely important that both ends of
the canaliculus are identified and reapposed. Sterile bandages
and antibiotic solution or ointment are kept on the wound until
the time of surgery. Multiple techniques have been developed
for adequate apposition of the severed ends of a canaliculus. It is
difficult to suture these directly, and consequently, most techniques utilize a metal, silicone, or polyester stent, such as a rod,
tube, or suture, which is threaded through both cut ends to act
as a scaffold over which the canaliculus can heal (Fig. 1-16). The
tissue around the canaliculus is then apposed with sutures. Recent
improvements in technique, particularly in isolating the ends of
the canaliculus, have significantly bettered the prognosis for a
successful reapposition.

Patching is not particularly important in the treatment of these
lacerations. However, the lids are sometimes sutured to each
other, to form solid support while the sutured lacerations are
healing. In addition, firm patching is important whenever a laceration, particularly a laceration of the canaliculus, occurs in an
infant. The patch will prevent him from disturbing the alignment
obtained by surgery.

A broad-spectrum antibiotic ointment is used to prevent infection. The affected eyelid is covered with an eyepatch for at least
24 hours, which may be removed, depending on the surgeon's
preference and the patient's sensitivity to light.

Burns

THERMAL BURNS. Thermal burns can occur from numerous
causes—explosion, hot molten metal, hot tar, steam, or fire.
Thermal burns of the lids are treated the same as burns anywhere else on the body.

Following a thermal burn, the capillaries dilate and the increased permeability allows the fluid to shift into the skin. The fluid is carried through the lymph system, with the excess fluid moving into the interstitial space and producing edema of the face and eyelids. Thermal burns will usually cause edema and hyperemia of the conjunctiva. If the lids are badly burned, there is considerable edema, and the eyes may be swollen shut.

Cold compresses are placed immediately over the burned areas. In industrial and emergency room cold packs are kept refrigerated for such purposes. If the tissue is contaminated, the nurse should wash off the lids and surrounding face with surgical soap and water before applying compresses. If pain prevents cleansing the injured tissue, systemic supportive therapy should be considered, since it will be necessary when definitive therapy is performed. Cold compresses are usually continued for 20 minutes or longer. All patients with burns should be examined by a physician and, if necessary, be transferred to the nearest burn center.

Cold compresses aid in constricting blood vessels, thereby causing less fluid to circulate in the damaged area. Also, the compresses are a comfort measure, reducing pain and lowering the skin temperature.

First and second degree burns of the eyelids require only symptomatic treatment. Antibiotic ointment should be used to cover any broken blisters. If the cornea or conjunctiva is involved cycloplegics are indicated and a combination antibiotic and steroid ointment will reduce inflammation. Third degree burns frequently cause marked lid edema. It may not be possible to examine the eye because of the lid edema. Antibiotic ointment and an appropriate dressing should be applied. Early skin grafting is indicated if scar retraction begins to occur.

One must be concerned about the globe of the eye in cases of severe burns. Even burns that do not appear to be extensive initially may cause some lid scarring, which could at a later date cause eye irritation because of changed configuration of the lid itself. Lidplasty at a later date would be indicated and would vary, depending on the problem.

A constant drip of an intravenous solution with an appropriate antibiotic and steroid can be directed onto the cornea and conjunctiva. A small plastic tube is inserted through the lid and positioned in the conjunctival fornix. A slow drip of solution can thus be delivered to the involved area. The same effect can be gained by taping a small tube to the lid margin.

Patients who have thermal burns of the face and eyelids are concerned about the loss of sight. Edema can be gross, causing the family to be quite emotional at seeing the patient for the first time postburn. The nurse should talk to the family before they enter the patient's room. An explanation of the amount of edema and why it occurs can be helpful to the family. The family is then prepared for the change in body appearance. A crisis such as an accident requires the nurse to spend some time assisting the family. At times, referral (a counseling agency) is necessary to help the family through the days of the patient's convalescence.

Explanations for procedures and what has occurred should be given to the patient. This is important even if the patient appears to be unconscious, as one never knows what the patient can hear.

CHEMICAL BURNS. Chemicals, whether acid or alkali, need to be washed from the skin completely, since they will continue to burn as long as they are in contact with the tissue. The eyes and the skin must be flushed copiously with water or saline.

In industry there are showers constantly running if dangerous materials such as acids or alkalies are being used. Also, there are water fountains with eight or more sprays which are used for eye washing and face washing. Workers are educated to run to these areas if an accident occurs.

The patient generally cannot hold his eye open, since the natural instinct is to close one's eye when something gets in it. Therefore, the patient or another fellow worker must hold the eyelid open, letting the water thoroughly flush the inside conjunctiva of both lids, the sclera, and the cornea. The flushing must be copious so that all foreign matter is removed.

Workers are told to wear safety glasses or goggles, when working with dangerous materials. Safety committees create posters, schedule meetings, discuss the necessity of proper action if an accident occurs, and are taught how to care for themselves as well as what to do for their fellow workers should an unforeseen occurrence arise.

After the eye is flushed with water, a steroid ointment is instilled. The eye is then patched. The patient should be transferred to a hospital for further evaluation.

If an explosion of oil or gasoline occurs, the eye should be

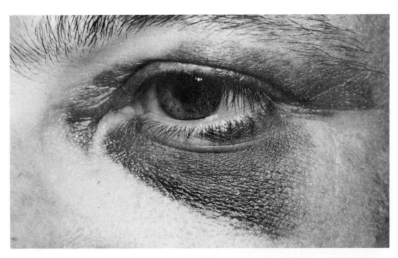

Figure 1-17. *Black eye. (Photo courtesy of Csaba L. Martonyi, Department of Ophthalmology, The University of Michigan Medical School.)*

irrigated copiously with saline or water. If the burn is so severe that the lid is damaged sufficiently to prevent it from closing, the cornea would be exposed and the lids must be sutured closed (tarsorrhaphy) or lidplasty must be performed.

Ecchymosis

The common black eye is caused by ecchymosis of the periorbital tissue (Fig. 1-17). There is no need for specific treatment other than to be sure that the eye itself has not been injured. It is well to remember that visual acuity should always be assessed before beginning any treatment or even cleaning the eye. This measure is taken to evaluate the patient's vision and also to protect the hospital or industrial company. The anterior chamber should be evaluated for depth and presence of blood, and the pupil should be evaluated for irregularities or differences in size when compared to the other pupil. Ecchymosis, or black eye, does not require treatment if no further damage to the eye has resulted. However, a thorough eye examination, including ophthalmoscopic evaluation, should be performed before the patient is discharged. Cold compresses relieve any local discomfort or edema that may result.

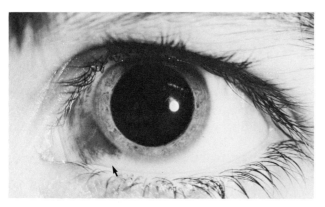

Figure 1–18. *Subconjunctival hemorrhage (arrow).*
(Photo courtesy of Csaba L. Martonyi, Department of
Ophthalmology, The University of Michigan Medical
School.)

CONJUNCTIVAL DISORDERS

SUBCONJUNCTIVAL HEMORRHAGE

Subconjunctival hemorrhage is a rather common condition. It appears as a bright red splotch on the area of the bulbar conjunctiva (Fig. 1–18). It is usually found in the interpalpebral fissure and usually adjacent to the limbus. It may be as small as 3 mm in diameter but may surround the cornea. If the hemorrhage is quite thick, it may be darker red, and may spread to cover a larger area during the first few days after its appearance. This does not mean that new hemorrhage has occurred, and the patient should be advised of this possibility. Despite its appearance, these hemorrhages never cause discomfort, and if discomfort is present, another cause must be found. The patient should also be advised that absorption will be slow and invariably takes one to two weeks.

Subconjunctival hemorrhage may occur after any trauma to the eye. However, most occurrences seem to be incidental and frequently are present on awakening. It may occur following stress such as sneezing or coughing, particularly in people with brittle blood vessels, blood dyscrasias, and diabetes. It is not necessary to evaluate a person system by system unless repeated episodes occur.

INFECTIONS

There are many agents causing conjunctivitis and many ways to classify them. According to the type of secretion, these agents are (1) catarrhal, (2) purulent, and (3) membranous.

Catarrhal conjunctivitis is signaled by a mucoid or mucopurulent discharge and marked by infected (bright red) and swollen palpebral conjunctiva. The bulbar conjunctiva is also infected but not usually to the extent of the palpebral. The discharge is often watery at first but soon becomes mucoid and then mucopurulent. Many bacteria can produce catarrhal conjunctivitis. The discharge is contagious.

Most catarrhal infections respond to topical sulfa preparations, but cultures should be performed if the condition is very severe or if initial therapy fails.

When this type becomes chronic it is usually caused by *Staphylococcus aureus, Streptococcus viridans,* or *Diplococcus pneumoniae.* The secretion becomes more purulent, and the symptoms are usually more severe at night.

Purulent conjunctivitis is most often caused by gonococci. Adult gonococcal conjunctivitis is associated with marked swelling, redness, and tenderness. The initial secretion is watery, but within two days the swelling is reduced and the secretions become purulent. The biggest danger is corneal ulceration and subsequent scarring. Once a diagnosis has been made, systemic and local therapy is indicated.

Ophthalmia neonatorum is the gonococcal conjunctivitis seen in the newborn. Inoculation occurs as the infant passes through the infected vagina. This was a serious cause of blindness until the instillation of silver nitrate solution (1%) was directed by law in most states in the 1930s and 1940s.

Other agents may cause purulent conjunctivitis, but it is rare for them to cause the severe reaction seen in gonococcal conjunctivitis.

Membranous conjunctivitis is so called because of the membrane that develops on the surface of the palpebral conjunctiva. This is a true membrane which causes bleeding when it is removed. It is almost always caused by *Corynebacterium diphtheriae.*

In addition, there are a few other typical clinical groups. *Follicular conjunctivitis* is diagnosed in the presence of many follicular-like lesions on the palpebral conjunctival surface. This is most often seen with virus infections and is also seen in the patient

with blennorrhea and trachoma. The secretions are often watery
and scant in the early stages of the infection.

Allergic conjunctivitis is associated with a watery mucinoid
discharge and itching (pruritus). Pruritus is not seen with the infectious types and is a good indication of allergy. Allergic conjunctivitis frequently becomes worse during the day and is better
at night. This does not occur with the other types of conjunctivitis.

A special type of allergic conjunctivitis, *vernal catarrh,* is often
seen during the warm weather. It recurs every spring and lasts
usually until the beginning of cold weather. Relief for allergic
conjunctivitis may be obtained by topical antihistamines or
steroids or both.

In any type of conjunctivitis, compresses are frequently applied
four times a day, or more often if possible. These compresses are
soothing as well as cleansing. Warm tap water can be used with
sterile 4 by 4 in. gauze squares or a clean washcloth. Because of
the infection, a different washcloth should be used for each eye.
The washcloth should be folded into fours, or quarters, so that
a different quarter is against the eye during any one application of
the compress.

LACERATIONS

Lacerations of the conjunctiva close readily. They are usually
healed solidly within 24 hours if the conjunctival margins are in
apposition. Even wounds into Tenon's capsule epithelialize readily
within a day, unless Tenon's capsule has prolapsed and prevented
apposition.

Complications such as a subconjunctival ecchymosis or intra-
conjunctival ecchymosis can occur. The primary treatment for
lacerations is to irrigate the eye with saline, give antibiotic eyedrops, and suture if necessary, pulling the ragged edges of the conjunctiva into apposition. The eye needs to be patched for comfort
only.

In the presence of any conjunctival laceration, however slight,
the possibility of a scleral laceration must be entertained. Thorough ophthalmologic evaluation is essential before the patient is
discharged.

FOREIGN BODIES

Conjunctival foreign bodies are common. They are usually not
uncomfortable unless they lodge under the upper lid, in which

case they rub the cornea each time the lid blinks. The foreign body is usually found in the sulcus that runs just above the inferior margin the full horizontal length of the lid.

These foreign bodies are usually visible with minimum magnification and can be easily removed with a moist cotton applicator. Care should be taken not to roll the applicator and damage the cornea by the foreign material sticking to the applicator and then being rolled into the eye tissue. As long as the cornea is not injured, topical antibiotic is not necessary. If a foreign body sensation is present and one is not found on the exposed conjunctiva or on the palpebral conjunctiva of the lower lid, the upper lid must be everted. The patient is placed in a sitting position looking at the floor. One then grasps the lashes firmly, places a cotton-tipped applicator on the center of the upper lid just below the skin fold, and simultaneously pulls the lashes out and up and presses in and down with the applicator (see Fig. 9–1). The tarsus will flip over and the lid will remain everted as long as the patient continues to look down. Merely asking the patient to look up will reposition the lid. If a foreign body is not discovered and suspicion still exists, the lid may be double-everted by everting the lid and then continuing to press downward with the applicator. This move will push the superior conjunctival fornix into view.

TUMORS

Nonmalignant

The most common tumor of the conjunctiva is the *pinguecula.* This is a small, yellowish, slightly elevated lesion seen in the interpalpebral fissure adjacent to the limbus. It may be on either temporal or medial side but is usually on both. It is more frequent as age increases. Histologically, it is formed from thickened sub-conjunctival hyaline and elastic tissue. It never becomes malignant and only rarely needs to be excised for cosmetic reasons.

Pterygium is a triangular fold of tissue that grows from the conjunctiva onto the cornea in the interpalpebral fissure. Although it is usually present on the nasal side, it may be present temporally. Its apex is firmly united to the cornea and it often grows far enough toward the center of the cornea to distort vision. If a pterygium appears to be progressing to the central cornea, it must be removed surgically before the central cornea is involved.

Papillomas have multiple appearances but usually are fleshy cauliflower-like lesions. They can be easily excised but may recur.

Leukoplakia and *intraepithelial epitheliomas* occur at the limbus. They have the appearance of opaque whitish plaques.

Nevi are common and should be watched for evidence of malignant change. Change in shape or color would warrant excision biopsy.

Malignant

All of the epithelial tumors (papillomas, leukoplakia, and epitheliomas) may develop into squamous cell carcinoma. These carcinomas usually remain superficial and can usually be excised.

Melanomas are usually black or gray. They are well vascularized and may be pedunculated. They are much less malignant than skin melanomas.

The possibility of a metastatic tumor to the conjunctiva, though rare, must be considered. Therefore, all suspicious lesions should be biopsied.

LACRIMAL SYSTEM DISORDER

The lacrimal system is seldom involved in infections unless the outflow channels are blocked. A purulent infection may develop in the lacrimal sac. This type of infection frequently occurs in newborns when the membrane across the end of the nasolacrimal duct in the nose does not separate. The tears accumulate in the lacrimal sac and usually become infected. Antibiotic drops or ointments will control the infection and daily pressure or massage over the sac will usually open such a blockage.

The massage is performed by having the mother take the side of her little finger or index finger and gently apply pressure by rubbing the sac. The lacrimal sac lies just in front of the infraorbital rim as it terminates on the temporal side of the nasal bone. During massage, the pus or infected material can be seen oozing from between the lids as it is forced backward and exudes from the punctum. If improvement does not occur by the age of 3 months, a probe can be slid through the canaliculus into the nose, breaking the membrane.

If blockage occurs in an adult, an operation must be performed to form a new channel. This is called a dacryocystorhinostomy. The lacrimal sac is exposed through a skin incision and its posterior aspect incised. A hole is cut through the nasal bone, and the nasal mucosa incised. The tissue of the sac is then sutured to the tissue of the nasal mucosa, forming a new drainage channel into the nose.

The incision is 2 to 3 cm in length, running diagonally down the side of the nose in the area over the lacrimal sac. Some physicians order warm compresses four times a day, to aid in comfort and prevent inflammation. While applying compresses the mother should note any redness or swelling that would indicate a cellulitis. An antibiotic ointment can be applied over the suture area as a prophylactic measure. If infection has been severe previous to surgery, systemic antibiotics may be ordered.

SELECTED READINGS

BOOKS

Bellows, J.G. *Contemporary Ophthalmology Honoring Sir Stewart Duke-Elder.* Baltimore: Williams & Wilkins, 1972.
Dunlap, E.A., (ed.). *Gordon's Medical Management of Ocular Disease.* (2d ed.). Hagerstown, MD: Harper & Row, 1976.
Zagora, E. *Eye Injuries.* Springfield, IL: Thomas, 1970.

ARTICLES

Gordon, D.M. Diseases of the eye. *Clinical Symposia* 14(4): 115–142, 1962.
Leopold, I.H. Anti-inflammatory agents in ophthalmology. *American Journal of Nursing* 63(3): 84–87, 1963.
Weinstock, F.J. Emergency treatment of eye injuries. *American Journal of Nursing* 71(10): 1928–1931, 1971.

CHAPTER 2 ─────────────

CORNEA AND SCLERA

ANATOMY

The outer coat of the eye is composed of a tough fibrous tissue approximately 1 mm thick. Roughly, it forms a ball with a slight bulge anteriorly. Its normal diameter varies slightly from person to person but measures approximately 24 mm anteroposteriorly and 23 mm laterally. The posterior five-sixths of the globe appears white and is called the *sclera.* The anterior bulge is called the *cornea;* it is transparent (Fig. 2–1).

The primary function of the cornea and sclera is to provide a rigid structure for the intraocular content. In addition, the cornea must maintain absolute transparency so that images can pass undistorted to the retina. The mechanism by which this occurs is not understood perfectly but it involves a balance between the passive movement of water into the cornea from the anterior chamber, evaporation from the epithelial surface, and an active metabolic elimination of water from the cornea. The integrity of the epithelium and endothelium is essential to this mechanism.

SCLERA

The sclera is composed of compact bundles of connective tissue arranged mostly parallel to the surface but running in all directions. There are multiple passages through the sclera to accommodate nerves and vessels as they pass to the inner structures. The largest of these openings is about 2.5 mm nasal to and slightly above the posterior pole of the globe. At this point, the sclera thins to a sieve-like membrane through which pass the retinal nerve fibers forming the optic nerve. This membrane is called the *lamina cribrosa.* It is about 1.5 mm in diameter (the diameter of the optic nerve) and is the weakest portion of the wall of the globe. Thus, when the intraocular pressure is elevated in glaucoma, it is here that the wall gives. Clinically, the lamina cribrosa can often be seen ophthalmoscopically in the normal eye as a stippled oval within the optic disc.

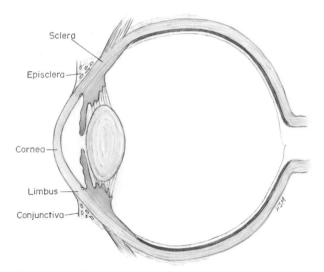

Figure 2-1. *Cross section of the eye.*

The sclera thins to about 0.3 mm at the muscle insertions, and the fibers of the muscle tendons intermingle with the scleral fibers. Anterior to the muscle insertions, the sclera thickens as it prepares to blend with the cornea. If the sclera is thin it will have a bluish appearance due to reflection from the dark choroid underneath. This is normal in newborns but will occur in any disease that thins the sclera.

The surface of the sclera is covered by a loose connective tissue called the *episclera,* which connects the conjunctiva to the sclera anteriorly. The sclera is almost void of blood vessels, but the episclera is relatively vascular. Anterior to the muscle insertions, the network of episcleral vessels becomes rather dense. It is these vessels that become engorged as a result of intraocular inflammation resulting in "ciliary injection" or "ciliary flush."

CORNEA

Epithelium

The cornea has five distinct layers (Fig. 2-2). The thin surface layer is composed of several layers of flattened epithelial cells. For all practical purposes, this layer is an extension of the conjunctival epithelium. The surface is very smooth and is in close apposition to a thin tough homogenous membrane called *Bowman's membrane.*

Epithelium – –
Bowman's membrane – –
Stroma – –
Descemet's membrane – –
Endothelium – –

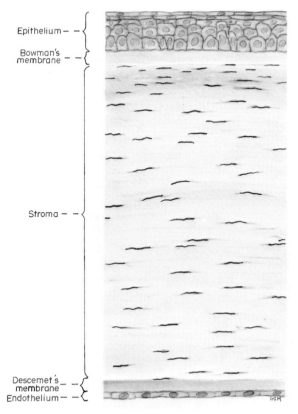

Figure 2-2. *Cross section, layers of cornea.*

Bowman's Membrane

Bowman's membrane, although usually described as a separate
layer, is actually part of the corneal stroma. It is composed of
tightly compacted connective tissue fibers, and its anterior surface
is exactly parallel to the anterior surface of the epithelium. Bowman's membrane forms a tough barrier to trauma or infection;
however, it does not regenerate if damaged, and a permanent
scar remains. Thus, trauma affecting only corneal epithelium will
not leave a scar but if the injury extends through Bowman's, a
scar will develop to the level of the injury.

Stroma

The *stroma* is composed of multiple lamellae of connective tissue,
all of which are parallel to each other and most of which are par-

allel to the surface. The fibrils composing the lamellae and the lamellae themselves are held together by a transparent cement substance. The stroma blends directly into the sclera. The major histologic difference between the two is that the connective tissue bundles are arranged much more regularly in the cornea. Traversing through the stroma between the lamellae is an interconnecting system of spaces or *lacunae.* These spaces function as lymph canals and, since the cornea does not have blood vessels, the lacunae provide nutriments from capillary loops at the corneal periphery throughout the stroma.

Descemet's Membrane

A very thin, structureless highly elastic layer forms the layer behind the stroma. It is called *Descemet's membrane,* and its elastic fibers extend into and beyond the periphery of the cornea to blend with the fibers forming the trabecular meshwork of the anterior chamber angle.

Endothelium

The innermost layer is a single layer of endothelial cells. This is known as the *endothelium.*

LIMBUS

A sulcus occurs at the periphery of the cornea where it joins with the sclera. This is known as the *limbus.* The conjunctiva and Tenon's capsule (the layer of orbital fascia that envelops the globe posterior to the cornea) join a short way behind the limbus and become adherent to the sclera at the limbus. The limbus is an important landmark for all types of anterior segment surgery (e.g., cataract, glaucoma).

EXAMINATION OF THE CORNEA AND SCLERA

SLIT LAMP

The slit-lamp biomicroscope or slit lamp is an instrument that permits examination of the surface of the eye under microscopic magnification (Fig. 2–3). It consists of a chin-rest to stabilize the patient's head, a multipowered microscope mounted on a movable platform, and a light source mounted on the same platform as

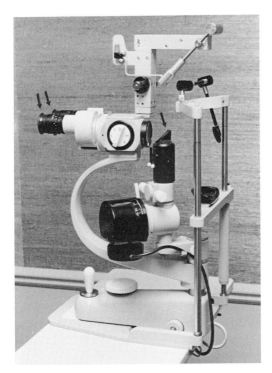

Figure 2–3. *Slit lamp. Binocular microscope (double arrow). Light source (single arrow). (Photo courtesy of Frank Flanagin, Associated Retinal Consultants, Detroit.)*

the microscope. The microscope and light source, therefore, move together and are controlled with a "joy stick", which controls forward, backward, and side-to-side movement. The power adjustment of the microscope enables the examiner to vary magnification from 5 times to 40 times, depending on the design of the instrument. The slit lamp receives its name because the width of its beam can be narrowed to a slit (Fig. 2–4). The advantage of doing this is that the narrowed beam of light (slit) can be aimed so that it will brightly illuminate only a narrow section of cornea or lens. The slit beam is angled from one side or the other of the microscope, and the examiner can then evaluate a thin slice or section of the cornea (or lens) at a time. This technique also enables the examiner to accurately localize the anterior-posterior position of any abnormality in the cornea anterior chamber, lens,

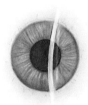
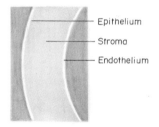

Epithelium

Stroma

Endothelium

A   B

Figure 2–4. *Slit lamp beam going through the cornea. A. Slit beam directed on cornea. Note curve of corneal light reflex compared to the straight light reflex on the iris surface just to the right. The slit beam is directed from the observer's left side. B. Appearance of slit of light through the cornea.*

or anterior vitreous. The slit beam is also helpful in determining the presence of cells in the aqueous. The amount of cells is a good indicator of the intensity of an iritis. An excellent comparison to this use of the microscope is the ability to see sediment floating in underwater swimming pool lights or fish bowl lights.

TOPICAL DYES

There are several topical dyes used to aid in the evaluation of superficial corneal defects. The one in most common use is fluorescein. In concentrations greater than 2%, it is a dark reddish orange color. However, when diluted it becomes a bright yellow-green and it temporarily stains the surface of the cornea where the epithelium has been removed or damaged. Fluorescein is available in solution and on fluorescein impregnated paper strips. It is difficult to maintain sterility of solutions, so paper strips are preferable. The technique involves application to the conjunctiva either by instilling a drop or by touching the conjunctiva with a moistened filter strip. After a few minutes, the excess dye is washed away with water or saline. Dye remains on the injured tissue. Fluorescein has an important place in evaluation of suspected corneal injury in emergency rooms, particularly if a slit lamp is not available. Fluorescein demonstrates a corneal abrasion when it is not otherwise noticeable with the naked eye or low-power magnification.

Rose bengal 1% and methylene blue 1% are also useful dyes but are more irritating than fluorescein. They do stain more deeply, and rose bengal must be irrigated quickly after instillation to prevent staining of normal epithelium.

DISORDERS OF THE SCLERA

INFLAMMATIONS

Inflammations of the sclera are uncommon. The sclera has a low metabolism and a poor blood supply so that most inflammations are only slowly progressive. Symptoms vary from mild discomfort to severe pain. The severity of the pain is not always commensurate with the intensity of the vascular reaction. There is usually tenderness to the touch.

Episcleritis involves the episclera and the superficial sclera. It is accompanied by intense vascular injection which may be localized or widespread and gives a reddish purple appearance to the area involved. The cause is usually obscure. In the past, the granulomatous infections, such as tuberculosis (in particular, leprosy and syphilis), were held accountable. Now, however, allergy and the collagen diseases, particularly rheumatoid disease, are considered most suspect. Treatment is dependent upon steroids, topical, subconjunctival, or systemic, as required.

Scleritis does not manifest the injection seen with episcleritis. There is pain, which often is severe despite the quiet appearance of the eye. In fact, there may be little external evidence that scleritis is present. A deep-seated pain and tenderness signal the disease. The causes and treatment are similar to episcleritis.

The result of scleritis or episcleritis can be scleral thinning. Patchy bluish areas indicate thinning and, if the sclera becomes very thin, the choroid may actually bulge outward. An outward bulge is called a *staphyloma.* Once a staphyloma has developed, danger of perforation is present. Treatment requires the grafting of a patch of preserved sclera or fascia lata to restore the integrity of the wall, but results are unpredictable and loss of the eye may ensue.

ACUTE INFECTIONS

Acute infections of the sclera are rare. They are almost always associated with trauma and often with retained foreign bodies. The most frequent cause in recent years has been postoperative infection of the silicone implants used in scleral buckling operations for retinal detachment. Cultures are routinely taken at the time of scleral buckling surgery, and intensive systemic and subconjunctival antibiotic therapy is often sufficient to control such infections. If immediate results are not achieved, it is necessary to remove the implant. Delay may lead to perforation of the globe and endophthalmitis.

DEGENERATIONS

Degenerations of the sclera occur with aging. The most common is called *senile hyalin plaque formation.* The condition occurs usually after age 50 but most often after 70, appearing as yellow-gray oval patches just behind the limbus in the palpebral fissure just anterior to the medial and lateral rectus muscle insertions. The *plaque* is actually thinned sclera containing a large amount of calcium salts. These do not progress and require no treatment.

INJURIES

Perforation and Laceration

The only serious scleral injuries are perforation and laceration. A perforation smaller than 2 mm in diameter usually seals itself spontaneously; any larger scleral break must be sutured closed. In the presence of a perforation from a long thin object, such as a dart or ice pick, the possibility of a through-and-through perforation with a posterior exit hole must be considered. An anterior laceration often extends under the conjunctiva, covering a large area. Consequently, when repairing such a laceration, the conjunctiva should be opened widely so that both ends of the wound can be positively identified. Closure can be effected with either interrupted or running sutures. Usually 5-0 or finer suture material is used, and either absorbable or nonabsorbable sutures are satisfactory. Funduscopic examination should be performed before or during surgery, and retinal holes treated with cryopexy, diathermy, or photocoagulation. If a retinal detachment is present, it may be possible to treat this at the initial operation. Blunt trauma can cause posterior lacerations without evidence of a penetrating wound anteriorly. If the vitreous is clear, the damage can be seen ophthalmoscopically. However, the vitreous is often filled with blood. This finding and the presence of a soft eye, usually with no recordable intraocular pressure, should alert the examiner to the possibility of a posterior rupture of the globe. Ultrasonography may be of help in establishing the diagnosis, but the visual prognosis even with adequate treatment is guarded.

Scleral Burns

Thermal and caustic burns can involve the sclera, but usually the cornea and conjunctiva take the brunt of these injuries. If the sclera is involved to a serious extent, the prognosis for salvaging the eye is poor.

DISORDERS OF THE CORNEA

INFLAMMATIONS OF THE CORNEA

Keratitis

Corneal inflammation (keratitis) can be caused by microbes, allergy, ischemia of the peripheral blood vessel arcade, and decreased lacrimation. The clinical appearance of the corneal lesion may be quite similar even with different causes. Consequently, these conditions will be discussed on the basis of their clinical appearance. The major symptom is pain, which may vary from as little as a foreign body sensation to severe discomfort. The vision may be unaffected if the visual axis is not involved, but vision is markedly reduced if dense central opacities are present in the cornea. Photophobia occurs frequently with the more severe forms.

The most common corneal inflammation is called *superficial punctate keratitis.* It has many different appearances, often subtle and usually recognizable only by slit lamp examination. The forms more commonly seen, their appearance, and causes are as follows:

1. Punctate epithelial erosions are tiny pits that become stained with fluorescein but otherwise may be very difficult to see even with the slit lamp. The most common causes are staphylococcal hypersensitivity secondary to conjunctival infection and mechanical or chemical irritants.
2. Punctate epithelial keratitis demonstrates gray-white flecks on the anterior epithelial surface. They are variable in size. The smaller lesions are caused by staphylococci, vernal conjunctivitis (an allergic conjunctivitis), and exposure. Coarser lesions are seen due to adenovirus, herpes (simplex and zoster), and superficial punctate keratitis of Thygeson.
3. Punctate subepithelial keratitis is gray spots just beneath the epithelium. The usual causes are herpes (simplex and zoster) and adenovirus.
4. Punctate stromal lesions may occur at any layer of the stroma. They tend to have fuzzy margins and are usually caused by herpes or trauma.

Most of these lesions are self limited and treatments can be symptomatic. If bacterial involvement is present, such as with staphylococcal lid infections, specific therapy should be instituted. Topical antibiotics (if needed) and steroids are usually sufficient to reduce discomfort. *However,* great care must be taken in prescribing steroids in a case of herpes; rapid worsening of the keratitis may occur unless an antiviral agent is given concomitantly.

Other Entities

STAPHYLOCOCCAL BLEPHAROKERATOCONJUNCTIVITIS. This condition demonstrates fine punctate epithelial erosions, usually on the lower third of the cornea. The site of the infection is probably the meibomian glands, and the conjunctival and corneal involvement is often sporadic as the chronic infection waxes and wanes. Treatment of the lid involvement is of primary importance. Warm compresses for several minutes followed by massage of an antibiotic ointment, such as erythromycin, along the lid margins with a finger or cotton tip applicator has been successful. This regimen is carried out morning and night for two weeks. Corticosteroids may be helpful in reducing the corneal symptoms but should not be used if a central corneal ulcer is present.

EPIDEMIC KERATOCONJUNCTIVITIS (EKC). This condition is an uncommon corneal disease caused by type 8 adenovirus. Initially, there are multiple punctate epithelial lesions, which, after one to two weeks, evolve into the typical coarse gray subepithelial lesions. These often are large enough to be seen with the unaided eye. The subepithelial lesions may remain for months. The onset is usually associated with a prominent conjunctivitis, photophobia, and discomfort. The acute symptoms subside much before the corneal opacities. Treatment with topical steroids appears to be the only effective method of limiting the size and number of opacities. There is a tendency for recurrence of the opacities upon cessation of treatment. Consequently, steroids are often prescribed at lowered dosages for months. Prophylactic treatment of EKC is particularly important because the disease is highly contagious. The largest outbreaks have been seen in busy eye clinics and institutions. All personnel should wash their hands after touching a patient suspected of having the disease, and any instruments used in the examination should be cleansed scrupulously.

PUNCTATE LESIONS. *Measles* and *mumps* may be associated with punctate lesions. Those seen with mumps are larger and often deeper. Supportive therapy and avoidance of bright light (to reduce photophobia) usually suffice. The lesions almost invariably disappear after several weeks.

Superficial punctate keratitis of Thygeson consists of large, grayish, elevated epithelial opacities that appear centrally and bilaterally. They may be associated with mild to moderate photophobia and discomfort. The cause is unknown. Steroids are effective in reducing the symptoms and the corneal lesions. However, since the disease may last for years, the lowest dosage should be used.

EXPOSURE KERATITIS. This condition can result from any cause that prevents adequate lid coverage of the cornea. From a nursing standpoint, it is particularly important to be aware of this possibility when caring for a comatose or unconscious patient. Primary treatment should be directed toward adequate corneal coverage by the lid. If the cornea remains exposed eye ointments or methylcellulose drops must be instilled regularly. If the cornea continues to dry out the affected eye must be patched. Narrowing the width of the palpebral fissure surgically (a tarsorrhaphy) is often adequate therapy. Otherwise lidplasty must be performed. Methylcellulose eyedrops or ointments are temporizing. If deep corneal ulceration or scarring develop, a corneal transplant would be indicated.

HERPES KERATITIS. This condition is probably the most common of the severe superficial corneal lesions. The danger is that the epithelial disease may progress and involve the stroma, forming a serious corneal ulcer. Herpes is a recurrent disease. Whenever the patient's resistance is lowered the corneal condition may recur.

The most characteristic appearance is that of a branching epithelial lesion called a *dendritic ulcer* (from the Greek *dendron,* for tree). The lesion may be very small or may extend across most of the cornea (Fig. 2-5). It is usually visible to the naked eye if stained with fluorescein. The vision is not affected unless the lesion falls within the visual axis. If the epithelium between the branches sloughs, the lesion is called a *geographic form* or *geographic ulcer.* The stroma is more likely to be involved but this lesion is still basically an epithelial lesion. Symptoms of epithelial lesions include mild to moderate irritation, lacrimation, and photophobia. Infrequently, there may be severe pain. Typically,

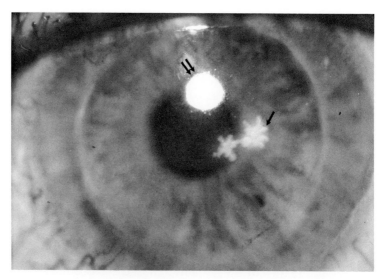

Figure 2–5. *Two confluent dendrites (single arrow) stained with fluorescein dye. (The double arrow points to the camera light reflex.) (Photo courtesy of Csaba L. Martonyi, Department of Ophthalmology, The University of Michigan Medical School.)*

the corneal sensation is reduced when compared to the other eye. This can be tested by touching a wisp of cotton to each cornea and observing the patient's blink response.

The first line of treatment for dendritic keratitis is the use of topical antiviral agents. Idoxuridine (IDU) was introduced in the early 1960s and has been demonstrated to be very effective. IDU is used as a 0.1% solution, one drop every hour during the day and every 2 hours at night. A 0.5% IDU ointment is available. The ointment, when used q.i.d., seems as effective as the more frequent use of drops. Seven to fourteen days of therapy are usually necessary, and the treatment should be continued for about one week after the epithelial lesion disappears to discourage recurrence. Before the introduction of antiviral therapy, mechanical removal of the involved epithelium was the primary treatment. This can be performed by anesthetizing the cornea with topical anesthetic and gently rubbing off the diseased epithelium. Some ophthalmologists recommend that this be performed before the institution of antiviral therapy and some save this treatment for those patients who do not respond to antiviral therapy. As new antiviral agents become available, (e.g., adenine arabinoside, trifluorothimidine, interferon, to name a few) fewer patients will be resistant to antiviral therapy.

Corticosteroids are definitely contraindicated in the treatment of epithelial herpes keratitis. Adequate documentation is available to show that corticosteroids increase the likelihood that the disease will involve the stroma—a development that signals a serious progression of the disease.

CORNEAL ULCERS

Herpetic Ulcers

Herpetic stromal keratitis is usually present to a mild degree in all cases of epithelial keratitis. It is recognizable by slit lamp as an area of mild anterior stromal infiltrate under the epithelial lesion. This usually clears slowly after the epithelial lesion heals. Occasionally, progression may result in deep stromal keratitis, which is often refractory to treatment and may lead to permanent scarring or even perforation of the cornea.

The treatment of stromal keratitis is complicated. Active virus is present in the stroma, but antiviral agents such as IDU alone have not been found to be beneficial. Occasionally, systemic steroids will be helpful. Topical steroids may be used but only in conjunction with repeated frequent slit lamp examination. Steroids should be used only with an antiviral such as IDU. Frequently, a penetrating corneal transplant is eventually necessary, but this should not be performed until the ulcer has been quiet for one year.

Disciform edema of the stroma is another less severe form of herpetic involvement. It appears as a round or oval area of stroma edema. Initially, the density of the lesion will be minimal but it may become quite dense (white). Most likely this condition is a hypersensitivity reaction. It may begin while the dendritic epithelial lesion is still present, or it may occur as long as months after the epithelial lesion has been resolved. Low doses of topical steroids are usually effective treatment. Antiviral coverage should be continued as long as steroids are used to discourage reactivation of an epithelial infection.

Bacterial and Mycotic Ulcers

The normal corneal epithelium is resistant to most bacteria and fungi. Injury to the epithelium will reduce the ability of the cornea to resist invasion and is the most common predisposing factor to the development of a bacterial or fungal ulcer. Injudicious use of corticosteroid eyedrops has also been implicated. The temptation is to regard minor corneal injuries, such as abrasions, foreign bodies, or drying by exposure, as being inconsequential. Although most of these lesions do heal rapidly, watching a minor lesion develop into a serious corneal ulcer is a most unpleasant experience.

Symptoms vary somewhat, depending upon the causative organism. There is always a grayish white to yellowish white opacity. It may be relatively small, 1 to 2 mm in diameter, or may involve most of the cornea. There is usually a grayish stromal infiltrate extending beyond the denser lesion. The eye may be markedly injected and a hypopyon may be present. On the other hand, there may be relatively little injection and pain.

Pneumococcal ulcers are the most common bacterial ulcers. A prominent hypopyon is usually present and is usually out of proportion to the severity of the infection. Chronic pneumococcal infection of the nasolacrimal tract should be investigated.

Pseudomonas ulcers are often explosive and may lead to perforation of the cornea within days. A hypopyon is usually present, and the eye appears markedly irritated. *Pseudomonas* has been discovered in eye solutions, particularly fluorescein solutions. Any eye medication suspected of being contaminated should be discarded. Some commercial fluorescein solutions have been demonstrated to be safe. If such a solution is not available, fresh solution should be procured daily or fluorescein paper strips should be used.

Staphylococcal ulcers are more common than has been emphasized in the past. They usually are rather indolent, are not usually associated with hypopyon, may be rather superficial and are often multifocal. They usually follow previous corneal insult such as exposure keratitis.

Gonococcal corneal ulcers are not common. However, the *Gonococcus* is one of the few organisms that will penetrate the unbroken epithelium. In addition, it has the characteristic of marked conjunctival exudate.

Fungal ulcers have certain characteristics, which, if present, are a help in diagnosis. Fungal ulcers are described as having a dirty gray color. There are often satellite lesions, and there may be branching at the margins. A history of injury by vegetable matter, such as a tree branch, or previous topical corticosteroid therapy, is often uncovered. Finally, if a bacterial cause cannot be demonstrated, a fungal origin should be suspected.

DIAGNOSIS. Corneal swabs and scrapings are used to make the diagnosis. Swabs should be taken from the conjunctiva and from the corneal ulcer, and should be cultured on appropriate media. Scrapings should be obtained using a small spatula under slit lamp observation. These scrapings should be cultured and smeared for appropriate staining. Although cultures are the most accurate method of obtaining a diagnosis, typical organisms will frequently be demonstrated on a stained smear. Proper antibiotic therapy may then be started a day or two earlier than if the diagnosis is dependent on culture.

TREATMENT. Topical or subconjunctival antibiotic therapy should be initiated as soon as culture material has been gathered. Broad coverage should be used if a diagnosis cannot be made by the smear. Therapy should include coverage of *Pseudomonas,* the most virulent gram-negative organism, and penicillinase producing *Staphylococcus,* the most difficult gram-positive organisms. Adjustments in coverage can be made when culture and sensitivities have been obtained.

Eyedrops are often used hourly around the clock until the situation is brought under control. Systemic antibiotics are not as effective as either the topical or subconjunctival routes. Subconjunctival antibiotics have proved to be extremely effective. Concentrations of subconjunctival antibiotic can be found in any ophthalmic pharmacology text or in the *PDR for Ophthalmology.* Subconjunctival injections may be uncomfortable in an inflamed eye. Usually the necessary concentration of antibiotic can be dissolved in 0.25 to 0.5 ml of solution. The injection is preceded by topical anesthetic (e.g., several drops of tetracaine) and subconjunctival injection of about 0.5 ml of 2% lidocaine (Xylocaine). The antibiotic can usually be injected in the area of lidocaine infiltration three to five minutes later. The use of tuberculin syringes with disposable ½-inch 27 gauge needles is the most convenient method. Care must be taken not to perforate the sclera as the needle is inserted under the conjunctiva.

Treatment of fungal ulcers is more complicated. Although many antifungal agents are known, most are very irritating, many are not very effective, and some are just not commercially available. Pimaricin (Natamycin) 5% suspension has a rather broad spectrum and is particularly useful against *Fusarium.* Nystatin (Mycostatin) has been somewhat helpful in treating *Candida* infections. Systemic therapy with any of the antifungals has not been demonstrated to be significantly beneficial. Often, repeated debridement is the most effective therapy.

In all cases of corneal ulceration leading to corneal scarring, penetrating or partial penetrating corneal transplantation may eventually be necessary.

Hypersensitivity Reactions

Marginal infiltrations or marginal ulcers are not uncommon lesions thought to represent a hypersensitivity infiltrate. They are white to yellowish in color and are present at the limbus on the corneal side but may be separated from the limbus by a narrow band of clear cornea. They may be multiple, and, if not round, will have their long axis parallel to the limbus. Their width usually is less than 1 mm. They are usually associated with a staphylococcal blepharitis or blepharoconjunctivitis. Treatment (topical antibiotics) should be directed at the chronic lid infection. Topical steroids will usually reduce the infiltrate; however, before initiating steroid therapy, one should rule out the possibility that the lesion is a herpes marginal ulcer, which lesion will be aggravated by steroids.

Phlyctenular keratoconjunctivitis appears as a whitish elevated abscess-like lesion at the limbus. It may progress onto the cornea and be accompanied by neovascularization. Lesions frequently recur; evidence of previous limbal scars will aid in the diagnosis. The lesions result from an endogenous systemic hypersensitivity. In years past, the most common cause was tuberculosis. Now, staphylococcal infections and coccidioidomycosis must also be considered. Topical steroid therapy will rapidly reverse the eye lesion. Appropriate systemic diagnostic efforts and therapy should be carried out simultaneously.

Vernal keratitis is a bilateral chronic recurring condition affecting children, usually boys, and seen in warm climates. Conjunctival involvement is always present, with papillary hyperplasia of the tarsal conjunctiva. Thick, stringy secretions are present over the conjunctiva and eosinophils usually can be demonstrated in scrapings. Often a limbal component will present round elevated mounds, called Trantas' dots. Extreme itching is the primary symptom, but photophobia may develop. Treatment consists of topical steroids, preferably in solution rather than suspension, and cool compresses. It may be necessary to move to a cooler climate.

DEGENERATIONS AND DYSTROPHIES

Pterygium is a fibrovascular overgrowth of the bulbar conjunctiva which extends across the limbus onto the cornea. Pterygium is invariably found at the horizontal midline, usually on the nasal side. It looks like a tongue of white tissue with its apex toward the center of the cornea. It is thought to be due to chronic irritation and is seen in people who spend a great deal of time outdoors. Treatment is unnecessary unless it approaches the visual axis. If this occurs, surgical removal should be carried out. The superficial cornea should be excised with the portion of the pterygium over the cornea. The lesion can be removed easily from its attachments to sclera. The conjunctiva is usually not sutured over the resulting defect at the end of the operation. Recurrences are common.

Arcus senilis is a condition common in the elderly, seen as a whitish ring or partial ring just central to the limbus and at most 1 mm wide. There is a clear space between the opacity and the limbus. It is due to a deposit of lipid material. If seen in the young or middle aged, the serum triglyceride level should be evaluated, although serum lipid levels are usually normal. Treatment is not necessary since the condition never involves the visual axis.

Band keratopathy, as its name implies, is a horizontal white or gray band extending across the central cornea horizontally in the midline. Classically, the band is 3 to 4 mm in vertical width and extends from 9 to 3 o'clock. There is hyaline degeneration and calcium deposition at the level of Bowman's membrane. This condition usually occurs following chronic uveitis or in a degenerating eye, though it may occur with parathyroid adenomas, Vitamin D toxicity, or renal failure. If there is potentially useful vision, removal can be accomplished by removing the epithelium and dissolving the material with a bath of the chelating agent edathamilcalcium-disodium (EDTA). A 0.01 or 0.05 m solution of EDTA is used as a corneal bath for fifteen or twenty minutes. This treatment has had good results. Any improvement may be temporary unless the general condition is resolved.

There are many types of hereditary dystrophies. Some affect the vision profoundly, others not at all. Dystrophies result in corneal opacification of different types. Dystrophies are often named by their clinical appearance (e.g., lattice, granular). Many are progressive, but some are stable. If the vision is seriously affected, a corneal transplant should be considered.

The most common dystrophy is called Fuchs' dystrophy. It is seen almost exclusively in the elderly and is caused by disruption of the endothelium leading to stromal and epithelial edema. The epithelial edema can often be controlled by topical hypertonic solutions (5% NaCl). If this is not effective, corneal transplant is often necessary.

ABNORMALITIES OF SIZE AND SHAPE

Microcornea is a condition in which the eyeball is essentially normal in size but the cornea is less than 10 mm in diameter. If the eyeball is small, the proper term would be microphthalmia. Eyes with microcornea are usually hyperopic and frequently develop glaucoma.

Megalocornea must be differentiated from congenital glaucoma. Megalocornea is defined as enlargement of the anterior segment, the cornea measuring greater than 13.5 mm. The anterior chamber is deep, and there is often iris atrophy. Although the intraocular pressure is normal in childhood, glaucoma secondary to lens dislocation may occur in adult life. The condition occurs in males and is bilateral.

Keratoconus is an uncommon condition in which the central cornea develops a noninflammatory conical protrusion (Fig. 2–6). The apex of the cone is just nasal and below the corneal midpoint. It is usually bilateral, often, though not always hereditary, and more common in females. The onset of symptoms usually occurs at puberty. The condition is slowly progressive but may become stationary at any time. The cone becomes more pronounced and the cornea thins. Vision is disturbed because of the irregularity of the eye's focusing system. In late stages, the diagnosis is easily made by looking at the cornea from the side or by holding the upper lid and observing the way the lower lid molds over the conical cornea as the patient looks down. In the early stages the abnormal refraction can be corrected by lenses, but contact lenses usually give a better optical result. Penetrating keratoplasty (corneal transplant) has a high success rate in this disease. This is the treatment of choice, if adequate vision cannot be obtained with contact lenses.

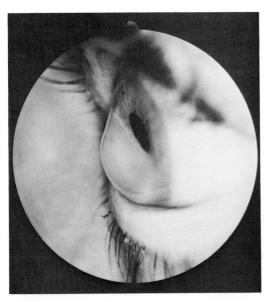

Figure 2–6. *Keratoconus. (Photo courtesy of Csaba L. Martonyi, Department of Ophthalmology, The University of Michigan Medical School.)*

TRAUMA

Abrasions

Abrasions, by far, must be the most common corneal injury. An abrasion is a disruption of the epithelium. The epithelium shows a remarkable rapidity for regeneration. Consequently, more often than not the patient will not seek medical care. Corneal abrasions may be quite uncomfortable because of exposure of nerve fibers in the epithelium and often are associated with photophobia, intense lacrimation, and iritis. The diagnosis is confirmed by slit lamp examination or by use of topical fluorescein instilled in the conjunctival fornix, by using either sterile drops or fluorescein impregnated filter paper moistened with a sterile solution. After one minute, the excess dye can be irrigated from the eye and any epithelial defect will stain bright green.

Since the epithelium usually heals within a day, treatment is necessarily short lived. Antibiotic eyedrops will guard against infection. Most of the discomfort occurs because of irritation by the upper lid as it rubs over the abraded area. A firm eye patch will immobilize the lid and usually relieve the pain. Rarely is an analgesic stronger than codeine necessary, and many people complain of no more than a foreign body sensation and require nothing more than reassurance. If the eye is still painful after it is patched, the patient may require bilateral patching to further limit eye movement. Occasionally, cycloplegics may be helpful in controlling iritis. Topical anesthetics are contraindicated, since they retard healing and give the patient an unwarranted sense of safety, which may lead to further trauma.

Recurrent corneal erosions are abrasions that recur spontaneously at the site of previous abrasions. It is thought that the epithelium does not adhere to the underlying Bowman's membrane following the initial injury. Recurrent erosions usually occur upon awakening in the morning. When the eyes are opened, a sharp stabbing pain and severe lacrimation occur. Most likely there is some adherence between the palpebral conjunctiva and the cornea because of less than ideal lubrication while the eyes are closed during sleep. Treatment is the same as that for an abrasion. However some ophthalmologists feel that the epithelium should be debrided and a tight pressure patch applied in hopes that the epithelial attachment will grow back stronger.

Any disruption of the epithelium, even if it is not abraded, may cause severe pain because of disruption of the nerve fibers in and under epithelium. Flash burns experienced by welders in industry are common injuries seen in emergency rooms. Flash burn is caused by ultraviolet waves and is the same as a sunburn. In fact, the same type of injury may be sustained from a sunlamp or the sun itself. (Snow blindness is caused by ultraviolet reflection from the snow.) The onset of symptoms may occur several hours after the injury just as it occurs with sunburn of the skin. The epithelium usually appears edematous and shows punctate staining with fluorescein dye rather than demonstrating an actual abrasion. Treatment is the same as for traumatic abrasion. The lesions heal quickly without sequelae. Cold compresses are soothing and relieve the discomfort. Tylenol gr X or Tylenol No. 3 (1 or 2 tablets) may be given for discomfort.

Another common cause of this type of lesion is the edema or abrasion caused by overwearing of contact lenses. These injuries are particularly common on holiday weekends or in resort communities when people break their normal routine and may stay up later than usual, exceeding their normal contact lens wearing time. Veritable epidemics may occur on the big football weekends in university towns. These injuries heal rapidly without visual loss, but antibiotic eyedrops should be prescribed to prevent development of a corneal ulcer. Since abrasions are so disabling when they occur, and since topical anesthetics will relieve the discomfort immediately, and since many patients know about the effectiveness of topical anesthetics, the temptation is sometimes great to give the patient a bottle of topical anesthetic to be used as needed for comfort. The danger is that further injury will go unnoticed by the patient as long as he continues to use the anesthetic and severe corneal ulceration may develop before it is diagnosed. If one does not plan to dispense anesthetic drops to such a patient, he should examine the patient without the use of anesthetic drops if possible. It is difficult to explain why anesthetic drops are not being dispensed when they have provided such obvious instantaneous relief.

Corneal foreign bodies constitute the most commonly seen eye injury in the emergency room. Certain workers (e.g., auto mechanics, grinding machine operators, power saw operators) are predisposed to sustaining this kind of injury. The injury is so common that it has given its name to the major symptom—*foreign body sensation.* Rarely, are the symptoms disabling and several days may pass before the patient seeks medical care. Ideally, the cornea should be examined with a slit lamp, although loupes and magnifiers are better than the naked eye. The examiner should always be alert to the presence of multiple foreign bodies. Also, if the history and symptoms are suspicious of foreign body, but only fine scratches and no foreign bodies are seen on the cornea, the upper lid should be everted and examined for foreign bodies.

Foreign Bodies

Corneal foreign bodies can frequently be irrigated from the corneal surface. If this fails, a moistened cotton tip applicator can be used. Care should be taken that the foreign body is not pushed along the epithelium causing more damage. Rolling the cotton tip applicator upon itself can cause ground glass to be embedded in the cornea.

Embedded foreign bodies should be removed by a physician. It is probably safer for him to remove the foreign body with a fine sterile spatula, called a foreign body spud. If it is not available, a hypodermic needle of almost any gauge will do. Iron and steel foreign bodies will leave a rust ring around the foreign body site. This can be removed using the spud, but battery powered hand drills about the size of a large dental drill are available and do a much cleaner job. Obviously, a topical anesthetic should be instilled before any attempt is made to remove an embedded foreign body. Antibiotic eyedrops should be instilled and continued for several days to discourage infection of the damaged cornea. An eyepatch should be applied at least until the anesthetic wears off.

Chemical Burns

Chemical burns of the cornea are treated exactly as conjunctival burns. (See Chap. 1, Burns, p. 21.) The emergency treatment demands on the spot irrigation with copious amounts of water. To delay while seeking consultation or assistance may be disastrous. Many plants have water fountains designed to irrigate the eye and face. Immersing the face in water and opening the eye under water is very effective. The primary concern is to remove all the foreign matter from the tissue of the eye. The eye must be held open so that it can be irrigated thoroughly with water or some bland solution.

Acid burns are quickly inactivated by the tissue so that most of the damage can be assessed soon after the injury. It is important to wash the eye copiously at the time of injury. Alkali burns continue to release toxic chemical components for long periods. It is important to remove all remnants of the alkali. Continuous irrigation with saline or steroid solution can be maintained by suturing a fine tube into the conjunctival sac. This fine polyethylene tubing is attached to an intravenous solution and thereby provides a continuous drip or irrigation. More recently, the action of collagenase, which is released from injured epithelial cells and has the ability to digest corneal stroma, has been studied. Chemicals such as acetylcysteine and penicillamine inhibit collagenase and are being used in these badly damaged eyes. Antibiotic therapy is also important. Often, corneal transplantation becomes the definitive therapy when the scarring process finally abates.

Lacerations

Corneal lacerations are a potential disaster to the eye. Often the globe is damaged beyond repair but even minimal lacerations may predispose to intraocular infection, cataract, corneal scarring, and irregularity. Some lacerations are so clean and small that they seal spontaneously. These should be treated with a rigid eyeshield and antibiotic therapy. Occasionally, a soft contact lens will be sufficient to oppose an otherwise leaking wound. Most lacerations require suturing. This is best done under an operating microscope with fine (7-0 or finer) suture. The type of suture (absorbable or nonabsorbable, running or interrupted) will vary according to the surgeon's preference. Maximum effort should be made to achieve the smallest scar since this will cause the least disruption of the final vision. If injuries to the conjunctiva, sclera, iris, lens, or even retina are present, attempts should be made to correct everything at the initial procedure. An eyeshield will be used at least at bedtime for several months depending on the size and strength of the wound. Cycloplegics and topical, systemic, or sub-conjunctival antibiotics are indicated. Appropriate tetanus therapy should be administered.

TUMORS

Most corneal tumors are extensions from the conjunctival tumors. They are usually superficial and can be removed by superficial keratectomy. Epithelial papillomas, intraepithelial epithelioma, and squamous cell cancer are the most common. In the cornea they are slow growing and rather benign.

Dermoid tumors of the cornea may occur as dense white lesions frequently at the limbus. They are like dermoid tumors elsewhere— congenital, rarely progress, and often do not effect vision. They can be removed and a corneal graft inserted for cosmetic or visual purposes.

SURGERY

Keratoplasty

Keratoplasty or corneal transplant surgery is the major form of corneal surgery. The procedure involves removal of diseased cornea and replacement with human donor cornea. Two basic procedures are performed: penetrating keratoplasty (full thickness graft) and lamellar keratoplasty (partial thickness graft) (Fig. 2-7). As instruments and techniques improve, the indications for lamellar keratoplasty become fewer.

The indication for transplant surgery is the presence of a scar

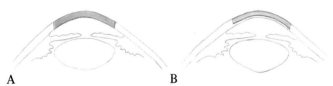

A   B

Figure 2–7. *Corneal grafts. A. Full-thickness. B. Lamellar.*

or irregularity sufficient to decrease vision materially. Attempts
should be made to evaluate the retina and the remaining ocular
components before proceeding. Ultrasonography, electroretinography, and related tests have allowed more thorough ocular
evaluation and more intelligent case selection. The potential for
visual improvement often depends on the type of scar rather than
the preoperative vision. Scars secondary to alkali burns do poorly.
Keratoconus scars do well.

Graft material is obtained from donors. Through a nationwide
system of eyebanks, eyes are collected, prepared, and stored for
corneal transplant surgery. The ideal donor material would be
from someone in early adulthood (25 to 35 years) who died of
an injury or an acute illness. The eyes are best enucleated under
sterile technique within an hour of death, although up to five
hours delay is acceptable if the eyelids have been closed and the
body refrigerated. The eyes are stored (corneas) in a tightly
closed container at 4°C. The eye should be used within two to
three days if it is to be used for a penetrating graft. Graft material for lamellar keratoplasty need not be as fresh.

Penetrating keratoplasties can be as large as the diameter of
the cornea or as small as 5 mm in diameter (Fig. 2–8). Grafts
smaller than 5 mm will not remain clear. The most common size
is between 7 and 8 mm because this size is usually large enough
to encompass the pathology, and more complications occur as the
incision gets nearer to the limbus.

The graft is removed from the donor eye first. The pupil is
constricted and the same trephine is used to cut a circular hole
in the host cornea. Usually, the trephine is centered on the cornea.
A cataract, if present, could be removed at this point in the
operation. If the eye is already aphakic, care will be taken to
remove any vitreous that may be in the anterior chamber and
prevent it from becoming incarcerated in the incision. Vitreous
can be removed with Weck Cell sponges and scissors or with a
vitreous suction-cutter machine. Usually four interrupted sutures

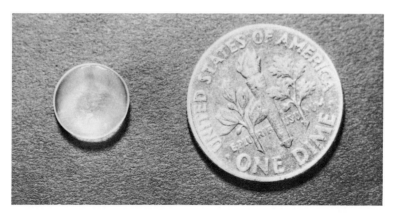

Figure 2–8. *Size of corneal graft versus size of a dime. (Photo courtesy of Csaba L. Martonyi, Department of Ophthalmology, The University of Michigan Medical School.)*

are then inserted, one at each point of the compass, to anchor the graft. Most surgeons then use a running suture to make a watertight closure, but others prefer multiple interrupted sutures (between 12 and 20) (Fig. 2–9). Finer sutures are constantly being developed and most surgeons now use 10–0 monofilament nylon. If a running suture has been used, the four interrupted sutures may be removed in several months but the running suture remains for a year or more (Fig. 2–10). A rigid shield is placed over the eye at the end of the operation. Topical cycloplegics and steroids are used until all uveitis resolves.

Lamellar keratoplasty has a place if the pathology is limited to the anterior stroma, or if the patient is uncooperative and there is fear that he might exert pressure on the eye after surgery. A partial thickness trephine incision is made and the donor material is then peeled away from the remainder of the cornea as one would peel an orange. The same thing is done on the host eye and the donor material is sutured in place. Although the optical clarity of a lamellar graft rarely matches that of a clear penetrating graft, the procedure has fewer operative and postoperative complications.

There are a few selected cases in which a keratoprosthesis may be indicated. Usually these eyes have dense scarring of the entire cornea, often with severe neovascularization. The prognosis for success of a penetrating graft in such an eye is essentially hopeless. Keratoprostheses are made out of nonreactive plastics, teflon, or silicone. They have a clear cylinder surrounded by a flat plastic cuff. A central penetrating trephine hole is cut and the surrounding

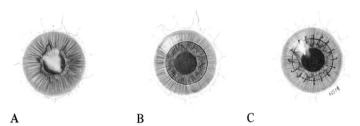

A   B   C

Figure 2-9. *Corneal transplant. A. Central opaque corneal scar.*
B. Recipient eye with central corneal button and scar removed.
C. Donor corneal graft in place with interrupted suture.

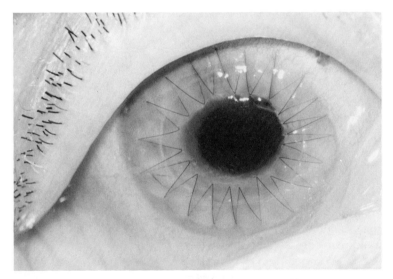

Figure 2-10. *Corneal transplant with running suture. (Photo courtesy*
of Csaba L. Martonyi, Department of Ophthalmology, The University
of Michigan Medical School.)

cornea is split so that the cylinder will extend through the trephine
hole and the cuff fit within the corneal lamellae. The visual results
occasionally are remarkable but the procedure is fraught with
complications and the long-term prognosis is poor.

Nursing care for patients having keratoprosthesis is similar to
those patients having corneal transplant surgery. However, the
prosthesis is kept clean by daily instilling a drop of solution used
to clean contact lens.

Evisceration and Enucleation

Severe insult of any kind may lead to serious degeneration of the entire eye. Although the globe may be very hard or mushy soft, the eye is irritated, painful, and blind. The term used to describe this condition is *blind painful eye,* and the treatment is enucleation or evisceration. Evisceration means removal of the inner contents of the globe but preservation of the sclera. Although removal of an eye is a major psychological adjustment, it is the only method of assuring relief of the severe pain, and it almost invariably promises a better cosmetic appearance.

An enucleation is begun by performing a 360° conjunctival incision, usually at the limbus. The rectus muscles are isolated and tagged with sutures before being removed from the sclera. The oblique muscles are then severed. The globe can then be lifted slightly out of the orbit and rotated to one side by grasping a stump of a muscle insertion. Some surgeons prefer to approach the optic nerve from the temporal side and some from the nasal side.

Most surgeons then apply a hemostat to the optic nerve to crush the blood vessels before cutting the nerve either with scissors or a knife. Some bleeding invariably occurs but this is usually controlled by pressing a gauze sponge firmly into the orbit. An artificial ball is then inserted into the orbit and the muscles tied over the ball. Tenon's capsule and conjunctiva are closed in separate layers with great care taken to be sure the implanted ball is well covered. Antibiotic ointment is placed into the conjunctival sac, a retainer inserted behind the lids, and a mild pressure dressing placed over the lids. Most surgeons leave the pressure dressing on for several days in an attempt to reduce postoperative edema.

The patient usually experiences little postoperative pain and can be discharged several days following surgery. A temporary prosthesis can usually be inserted between the lids within a week but a tailor-made prosthesis will be designed by the prosthesis maker. Prostheses are made of plastic and can be painted to match the normal eye almost perfectly. These prostheses are generally tolerated very well. The patient soon learns to remove it for cleaning. Ophthalmologic evaluation of the socket should be performed at least annually, since erosion of the implanted ball may occur.

Eviscerations are performed less frequently than enucleations if
for no other reason than a complete pathologic specimen is not
available. Although some surgeons feel that eviscerations give a
better cosmetic result, newer implants and meticulous technique
appear to give about equally satisfactory results with either
procedure. Eviscerations are performed by removing the cornea
and scooping out the contents of the globe. A gauze sponge is
then used to scrub as much pigment from the inner scleral wall
as possible because it is felt that retained pigment may predispose to sympathetic ophthalmia. An artificial ball is then inserted inside the globe and the anterior surface covered either
by resuturing the cornea over the opening, by covering the opening with Tenon's capsule and conjunctiva, or by doing both.
The remainder of the postoperative care is identical to the care
following enucleation.

If these procedures are performed at the proper psychological
moment, patients are very grateful for the relief of pain and the
much improved cosmetic appearance. However, surgery is a
psychological letdown. The patient keeps hoping for a recovery
and these procedures are final; there is no longer hope for functional vision. Patients need emotional support to prepare them
for surgery and to accept the postoperative outcome.

Preoperative nursing care is routine. Postoperatively, patients
return from the operating room with a pressure dressing over the
affected eye. Vital signs are monitored until stable. Patients
generally may be up on the first postoperative day. Emotional
support is one of the important aspects of their immediate postoperative care. Patients are discharged approximately 3 to 5 days
postop. The eye is patched. They return in approximately ten days
to visit the surgeon. At this time or shortly thereafter they receive
their prosthetic eye. Patients are taught how to care for their
eye and socket. (See Chap. 10, Cleaning Eye Prosthesis, p. 275.)
It is important to remember that the prosthesis is a foreign body,
so that the socket should be irrigated frequently and the prosthesis removed daily for cleaning.

Preoperative Nursing Care

The patient who is to have a corneal transplant generally has his
name put on a waiting list for the cornea. The waiting time,
once one's name is on the surgery waiting list, is six to eight
weeks. However, patients may wait for months to a year to be

placed on the surgery waiting list. Therefore, the patient may have only 24 hours notice or less that he is to be admitted to the hospital for his corneal transplant. Transplants that are performed 24 hours or less after obtaining the cornea from the donor have the best chance of obtaining functional vision. The patient, while he has been waiting weeks to be notified of his surgery, finds himself uneasy and rushing to prepare for his departure to the hospital. He is anxiously concerned about the success of surgery. While the patient has had poor vision and surgery will not make his visual function less functional, his concern turns to hoping for a perfect graft. Usually the fact that the time has arrived for surgery makes the patient uneasy. The 8- to 12-week wait for the corneal graft does not eradicate the anxiety that comes to surface when surgery is imminent.

Routine laboratory work is done preoperatively as soon as the patient is admitted. This does cause some added anxiety, as many things are being carried on at one time, with relatively short explanations to the patient. The admission, the laboratory work, and the preoperative nursing care all make for some tense moments for the patient. Needless to say, a quiet but efficient manner is rather soothing to the patient.

The patients also receive glycerin (Osmoglyn), which reduces edema of the cornea and lowers intraocular pressure. The usual oral dose is 1 gm/kg body weight mixed with tart juice one hour preoperatively. Diazepam (Valium) 5 or 10 mg orally is given 1½ hours preoperatively. It is used as a preoperative sedative, and if general anesthesia is used it is a helpful preinduction medication.

Patients should be told if they will be awake throughout the procedure. It is well for them to know that the local anesthetic will burn and be uncomfortable momentarily when the material is injected. The patient should be told of the importance of not jerking or moving during the surgery. While some patients fall asleep, they can or may awake with jerky quick movements, while others awake quietly. Quick or unexpected movements on the part of the patient could be disastrous. It is probably well for the circulating nurse or the surgeon to check with the patient as to how he is feeling and to give him a little progress report of the surgery. This type of checking before critical times in the surgical procedure might be the difference between a successful and an unsuccessful corneal graft result.

Preoperatively, the patient receives miotic eyedrops if the patient will not be having a lens extraction or a vitrectomy.

Pilocarpine is frequently used to constrict the pupil. The patient receives one drop every five minutes times two drops. If the patient will be having a lens removed or if a vitrectomy is planned, the eye is dilated with a mydriatic-cycloplegic eyedrop. Atropine 1% or cyclopentolate (Cyclogyl) 1% are frequently the drops of choice for dilatation. The patient receives one drop every five minutes times two drops.

Postoperative Nursing Care

Patients who return from the operating room need to have their vital signs monitored. If an intravenous infusion is running, it is discontinued when infused.

The patient is permitted out of bed to the bathroom with assistance when fully recovered from anesthesia. Generally patients receive liquids to a soft diet for their first postoperative meal. They may have fluids and return to a regular diet as tolerated.

Patients may be out of bed on the first postoperative day, but generally walk only to a chair to sit for a brief period or are up to go to the bathroom. Tylenol No. 3 one or two tablets or meperidine (Demerol) 50 mg intramuscularly can be given for discomfort. An antiemetic is ordered for nausea or vomiting if necessary. Generally, nausea and vomiting are not a problem.

The patient returns from the operating room with the operated eye patched and a metal or a plastic shield applied for added protection. The patient generally wears the patch and shield for the duration of the hospital stay. The shield is worn at night for approximately three to four months. However, both patching and length of time for wearing the shield vary with the individual surgeon's preference.

The eye is kept dilated with atropine sulfate 1% t.i.d. Prednisolone sulfate drops, one t.i.d. is the steroid used to prevent inflammation and graft rejection. Instillation of a sulfa drop such as sulfacetamide sodium, one drop t.i.d., is a prophylactic measure. Patients are discharged with these three drugs. Eyedrops are instilled for a few months after surgery. Generally, the eye medications are tapered off beginning four to six weeks after surgery.

Patients are discharged five to seven days postoperatively. They return to visit the doctor one week after discharge. Vision varies after surgery from count fingers to fairly acceptable vision. Patients should be told that functional vision is frequently not attained until the sutures are removed, approximately one year from the day of surgery.

Discharge teaching is similar to that for the patient having cataract extraction. (See Chap. 5, Hospital Procedure.) The patient should avoid any stress on the suture line such as bending over at the waist, or avoid any activities that would cause an increase in intraocular pressure. Lifting heavy objects or moving heavy furniture can cause stress on the suture line and, therefore, should be avoided.

Patients are told to assess their eye at approximately the same time each day for corneal graft rejection. Signs and symptoms are redness of the eye, increased discomfort, or change in far vision. Patients should realize that the graft is never a part of their own body and can, therefore, be rejected at any time. Some patients have had graft rejection years after their transplant surgery. Therefore, the patient for the rest of his life must assess his eye for symptoms of graft rejection.

Contact Lenses

Contact lenses, as the name indicates, are corrective lenses that rest on the cornea. Although most contact lenses are probably sold because of their cosmetic appeal, they have definite medical values. They are useful in cases of large refractive errors, particularly when there is a great difference in the refractive error between the two eyes. The larger plus (farsighted) glasses cause magnification (e.g., postoperative cataract glasses) and the larger minus (nearsighted) glasses cause minification. This optical fact of life cannot be adjusted with regular glasses. Contact lenses do reduce the amount of size differential. Thus, a person who has a large difference in the glasses correction between the two eyes will be able to cope with the difference in image size if he wears a contact lens on the eye with the greater correction. He may, of course, wear contact lenses on both eyes. Contact lenses also reduce the effect of corneal irregularities and may improve vision significantly. Because the contact glass curves over the cornea, it provides less peripheral distortion than does a spectacle glass.

There are two types of contact lenses—hard (acrylic plastic) and soft. At present the hard lenses give better optical definition (better vision) but they are more difficult to wear, and wearing time usually does not exceed 12 to 14 hours. If a person's normal wearing time is exceeded, the cornea may become edematous or abraded and painful. Most hard lenses are corneal lenses. Their diameter is less than the corneal diameter (usually about 9 mm) and they ride on the precorneal tear film.

There are scleral hard contact lenses that have a larger diameter than the cornea and rest on the sclera. They form a chamber in front of the cornea, which must be kept full of fluid. Scleral lenses are less comfortable and harder to wear than the corneal lenses.

Soft contact lenses are very pliable. They are much more comfortable, as a general rule, than hard lenses. They can often be worn for days at a time. They do not have the same optical clarity as hard lenses but they are much improved compared to the initial lenses brought out in the early 1970s. They extend onto the sclera and are so thin that it may be difficult to tell that a person is wearing lenses. Soft contact lenses have achieved a place because they are more comfortable and they can be used therapeutically to seal corneal perforations and to cover certain corneal ulcerations.

SELECTED READINGS

BOOKS

Bronson, N. R., II, and Paton, R.T. *Advances in Keratoplasty: A Symposium Sponsored by the Eye-Bank for Sight Restoration and the Southampton Hospital.* International Ophthalmology Clinics. Boston: Little, Brown, 1970.

Casey, T. A., (Ed.). *Corneal Grafting,* New York: Appleton-Century-Crofts, 1972.

Donaldson, D. D. *Atlas of External Diseases of the Eye.* Cornea and Sclera. St. Louis: Mosby, 1971. Vol. 3.

Dunlap, E. A., (Ed.). *Gordon's Medical Management of Ocular Disease* (2d ed.) Hagerstown, MD: Harper & Row, 1976.

Ellis, P. *Ocular Therapeutics and Pharmacology* (5th ed.). St. Louis: Mosby, 1977. Pp. 117-118.

Grayson, M., and Keates, R. H. *Manual of Diseases of the Cornea.* Boston: Little, Brown, 1969.

Wade, A. (Ed.). Iodoxuridine. In W. Martindale (Ed.), *The Extra Pharmacopeia* (27th ed.). London: Pharmaceutical Press, 1977. Pp. 912-914.

ARTICLES

Boyd-Monk, H.   Helping the corneal transplant patient to see again. *Nursing '78,* pp. 47–51, Feb. 1978.

Breinin, G. M., and DeVoe, A. G.   Chelation of calcium with edathamil calcium-disodium in band keratopathy and corneal calcium affections. *AMA Archives of Opththalmology* 52(12): 846–851, 1954.

Levenson, L., et. al.   Corneal transplantation. *American Journal of Nursing* 77(7): 1160–1163, 1977.

CHAPTER 3 —————————————

IRIS, CILIARY BODY, AND ANTERIOR CHAMBER

ANATOMY

IRIS

The *iris* gives color to the eye. A thin curtain, it springs from the ciliary body but also is attached to the sclera about 2 mm behind the corneal limbus, and it hangs freely. It has a central round opening, the pupil. The central iris rests against the anterior surface of the lens. When the lens is absent, the iris moves posteriorly, deepening the anterior chamber and the iris floats in the aqueous.

The iris is made up of three layers. The two anterior layers are mesodermal in origin and form the stroma. It is a loose organization of connective tissue interspersed by vessels and a variable amount of pigment. The deepest layer is of neuro-ectodermal origin and is actually two layers of dark pigment cells. The darkness of the iris depends on the amount of pigment in the stromal layers. Blue eyes have very little pigment; brown eyes have a great deal.

Two important muscles are present within the stroma: the sphincter and the dilator. The sphincter is a flat 1 mm wide ring of muscle that surrounds the pupil margin. When it contracts, the pupil constricts. The dilator muscle is a very thin layer of radially arranged muscle fibers that lie in the posterior portion of the stroma, fuse with the sphincter muscle centrally and attach in the ciliary body. The dilator fibers are processes of the more anterior pigment cell layer.

The primary function of the iris is to control the amount of light reaching the retina. Thus, the sphincter and dilator work together to vary the pupil opening, constricting it in bright light and dilating it in dim light.

The dilator muscle is stimulated by the sympathetics and thus dilates whenever the person is excited and adrenalin is released. The sphincter is stimulated by the parasympathetics. Appropriate drugs will have their effect on the pupil. Thus, the pupil will be dilated by adrenalin-like (phenylephrine [Neo-Synephrine]) or acetylcholine (parasympathetic) blockers (atropine, homatropine, cyclopentolate [Cyclogyl], tropicamide [Mydriacyl]). On the other hand, it will be constricted by acetylcholine-like (pilocarpine, carbachol) or anticholinesterase (phospholine iodide, demecarium bromide [Humorsol]) drugs.

CILIARY BODY

The *ciliary body* extends posteriorly from the iris and connects with the choroid. It has two major parts: the ciliary muscle and the ciliary processes. The ciliary muscle contains two muscle groups. The outermost fibers run in an anterior-posterior fashion. They originate at the scleral spur at the anterior chamber angle and extend posteriorly into the outer layers of the choroid. The inner portion is comprised of fibers arranged in a circular fashion just behind the iris. Contraction of the ciliary muscle causes the ciliary body ring to reduce in size. This contraction loosens the zonules supporting the lens and allows the lens to become more convex. Thus the ciliary muscle controls the lens focus. The use of parasympathetic blockers (atropine) not only dilates the pupil but paralyzes accommodation, blurring the near vision.

There are approximately 70 ciliary processes—narrow folds running in a meridional fashion (anterior-posterior) and lying on the inner side of the ciliary muscle. They consist almost entirely of blood vessels, most of which are veins.

The aqueous fluid is produced by the ciliary processes. It enters the anterior chamber through the pupil and leaves the eye by outflow channels in the anterior chamber angle (Fig. 3–1). The aqueous has two basic functions: to supply some nutrients to the cornea, lens, and vitreous, and to maintain pressure in the eye.

ANTERIOR CHAMBER

The *anterior chamber* is bordered by the cornea anteriorly and the iris and lens posteriorly. The anterior chamber angle (Fig. 3–2) is an extremely important structure; abnormalities here may reduce aqueous outflow, leading to elevated intraocular pressure and glaucoma. The angle is formed at the site of the origin of the iris from the ciliary body. A small lip of sclera extends toward the anterior chamber at the apex of the angle. This lip is called the *scleral spur.* The ciliary body inserts on the posterior aspect of the scleral spur and the apex of the anterior chamber angle is at

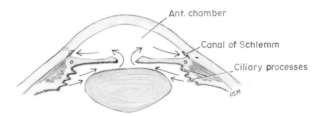

Figure 3-1. *Aqueous fluid.*

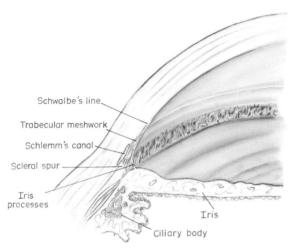

Figure 3-2. *Anterior chamber angle.*

the anterior edge of the scleral spur. A small furrow is present just anterior to the body of the scleral spur. This space has within it a meshwork, the *trabeculum,* which allows aqueous to escape into an irregular tubular structure that forms a ring around the anterior part of the globe at the apex of the furrow. This tubular structure is called *Schlemm's canal* which in turn has multiple exit channels that empty into veins within the sclera and the episclera. Thus, the aqueous eventually is absorbed into the general circulation.

EXAMINATION OF THE ANTERIOR CHAMBER

GONIOSCOPY

The anterior chamber angle and its structures cannot be seen by looking directly at the eye, because the angle is positioned posterior to the periphery of the cornea, tucked behind the anterior extension of the sclera. This zone can be seen with a special corneal contact lens, or gonioscope. A microscope, usually the slit lamp, is used to obtain magnification.

TONOMETRY

The tonometer is the instrument used to measure intraocular pressure (also referred to as *intraocular tension* or *tension*). Several types of tonometers have been developed. They all depend on indentation of the globe and a measurement of the force necessary to achieve indentation. The scale reading of the instrument is then converted to the actual pressure in millimeters of mercury by the use of experimentally developed conversion charts. Some of the newer instruments are calibrated to read in millimeters of mercury. The oldest and most popular tonometer now in use is the *Schiøtz tonometer.* It has a curved footplate, which is placed on the anesthetized cornea. A piston moves through a hole in the footplate and indents the cornea. The amount of the indentation registers on a scale and a conversion table is used to convert scale units into millimeters of mercury. The instrument must be held vertically and the patient should be looking straight up. It is essential that the instrument be clean so that the piston does not bind within its shaft, invalidating the reading. The examiner must hold the patient's eye open. It is important that the patient's lids be relaxed, otherwise the pressure exerted by squeezing the lids will increase the intraocular pressure (see Fig. 9–9).

The *applanation tonometer* uses a flattened plastic cone to flatten a small area of cornea. Fluorescein dye and blue light are used to observe the flattening. Spring tension is regulated while observing the plastic cone with a slit lamp (Fig. 3–3). The end point is reached when two half circles inside the cone are seen to match. The pressure is read directly from the spring tension knob.

Several instruments have been introduced in recent years. Some do not require anesthetic. One uses a puff of air without actually touching the cornea—called the *noncontact tonometer.* These newer instruments have proved to be accurate but they are significantly more expensive. Their use has been increasing because patients may be tested more quickly and because testing can be performed while the patient is in the sitting position.

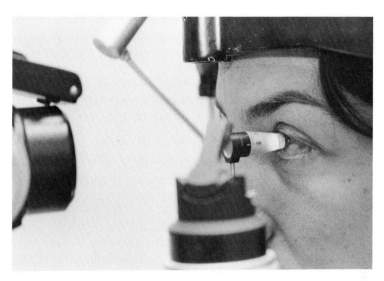

Figure 3–3. *Applanation tonometer. (Photo courtesy of Frank Flanagin, Associated Retinal Consultants, Detroit.)*

DISEASES OF THE ANTERIOR CHAMBER

GLAUCOMA

Glaucoma is a condition in which the intraocular pressure has become elevated sufficiently that it has caused structural or functional damage to the eye. Understanding of the term is complicated somewhat because it has been used to describe the condition wherein the intraocular pressure is raised to a level known to cause glaucomatous damage, even though no damage has occurred. In fact, the term is used when the pressure is controlled in the normal range by medication if the pressure would be at a dangerous level without medication.

Thus in normal usage, glaucoma usually refers to a condition in which a person is taking medication to reduce what has been judged to be abnormally high intraocular pressure to the normal range. In most instances, no permanent ocular damage has occurred and never will if treatment is continued. The disease, however, is chronic. Medication will not cure it, and treatment will usually be necessary for the remainder of the patient's life. Surgery, on the other hand, often is curative.

Diagnosis

The diagnosis of glaucoma is not difficult if the patient is seen
in the late stages of the disease. Demonstration of elevated intraocular pressure, typical visual field defects, and excavation of
the optic disc will confirm the diagnosis. However, the objective
in treating glaucoma is to begin treatment before serious ocular
damage occurs. On the other hand, treatment is inconvenient and
should not be initiated without strong evidence of the elevated
pressure of glaucoma.

INTRAOCULAR PRESSURE. Normal intraocular pressure is considered to be approximately 15 mm Hg. Pressure >21 mm Hg is
considered suspicious, and pressure >24 mm Hg is generally considered abnormal. In addition, it is unusual for a difference of
more than 3 mm Hg to occur between the two eyes if they are
normal. There is a normal diurnal pressure variation of 3 to 5 mm
Hg. The pressure is highest in the morning before arising and
lowest in the late evening. In glaucomatous eyes, the variation
may be as much as 25 mm Hg.
    It is well known that some eyes will tolerate pressures >30 mm
Hg for long periods without apparent damage. Other eyes may develop structural changes from glaucoma, with intermittent pressures often in the 20s.
    A high index of suspicion is essential if early diagnosis is to
be made. Tonometry should be a part of every complete adult
eye examination, and generalists should be encouraged to include
tonometry in their general physical examination. Approximately
one-third of glaucoma patients have a family history of glaucoma.
This information should be noted in the assessment. Patients
with intraocular pressures in the low 20s should be seen often
enough to establish the maximum intraocular pressure. Repeat
examinations at least annually would then be required. If the
pressures run in the high 20s provocative tests should be considered.

VISUAL FIELD. Central visual fields should be performed in all
glaucoma suspects. The central field chart or tangent screen is a
1 meter by 1 meter flat board placed 1 meter in front of the
patient. The target size is usually between 1 mm and 10 mm, depending on the patient's vision. The 3 mm target is probably the
most common size for initial screening. Different size targets
are used to demonstrate the "density" of a field defect. Some

defects may be absent with large targets and are considered less dense than those that are present to large and small targets. Central fields cover about 50° of the patient's vision—that is, 25° in each direction from the center of fixation. Each eye is tested separately.

Visual field changes in uncontrolled glaucoma are progressive. The initial sign is a superior and inferior enlargement of the normal blind spot, the so called Seidel's sign. This may progress to a scotoma which extends from the disc to the periphery. This is called baring of the blind spot. Arcuate scotomas (blind areas in the field of vision) which begin at the blind spot and extend either superiorly or inferiorly in an arc-like configuration beyond the center of fixation to the horizontal meridian on the opposite side, are another classic sign of glaucoma. These are called Bjerrum's scotomas (Fig. 3–4). When Bjerrum's scotoma extends to the nasal horizontal meridian, it often shows a wider scotoma superiorly than inferiorly. This will give a step-like configuration of the scotoma pattern if the recording chart is laid on its side. This is known as Rönne's nasal step.

These three visual field signs—Seidel's sign, arcuate scotoma (Bjerrum's scotoma), and Rönne's nasal step are classic diagnostic signs of glaucoma. Continued progression will lead to gradual reduction in the peripheral field until only a small central field remains. The patient's central vision may be very good until the final stages when all vision will be lost.

AQUEOUS OUTFLOW. Tonography is a technique used to study the outflow of aqueous from the anterior chamber. Since most cases of glaucoma are secondary to reduced outflow, the information is helpful in evaluating borderline glaucoma. Pressure on the eye increases the normal aqueous outflow. This outflow is measured by repeated tonometric readings. An electric indentation tonometer, similar to the Schiøtz tonometer, has been connected to a recording drum to allow continuous recording of the intraocular pressure. This tonometer is rested on the cornea for four minutes.

A coefficient of aqueous outflow is calculated from the record obtained. Normal eyes have a coefficient of aqueous outflow of 0.28 ± 0.05. Only 2.5 percent of normal eyes have an outflow of 0.18 or less. Another indicator obtained from the tonography tracing is the Po/C value. This is calculated by dividing the initial intraocular pressure (Po) by the coefficient of outflow (C). Only

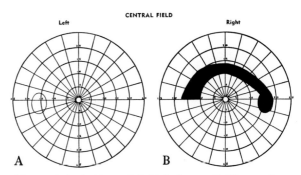

Figure 3–4. *A. Normal field, left eye. B. Bjerrum's scotoma, right eye.*

a small percent of normal eyes have a Po/C ratio of 140 or higher.

When the diagnosis remains unclear, provocative tests may be helpful. These tests are not always reliable. In addition, they carry some risk of causing serious elevation in the intraocular pressure, which may require prompt therapy. They should be performed under the supervision of an ophthalmologist experienced in handling such problems.

PROVOCATIVE TESTS. Provocative tests are not necessary for all glaucoma suspects. They should be considered for eyes which have pressures over 22 mm Hg, outflow below 0.18, and Po/C over 100, without other signs. They should also be considered in eyes with suspicious visual field changes or optic disc changes in the absence of other diagnostic signs.

Water Drinking Test. The water drinking test is performed by having a fasting patient drink one liter of water as rapidly as possible (within two to five minutes). The test is performed in the morning. The pressure is taken before and again 45 minutes after the water is ingested. A rise in pressure of ⩾7 mm Hg is considered indicative of glaucoma. Normal eyes usually show a rise of 3 to 5 mm Hg. Tonography may be performed at the end of 45 minutes. Abnormal tonographic calculations (<0.18 or Po/C>100) would strongly suggest glaucoma.

Corticosteroid Tests. Topical instillation of corticosteroids, if given for a sufficient period of time (several weeks) on a regular basis, may cause elevation of intraocular tension and decrease of the facility of outflow. A rise in tension > 7 mm HG and a Po/C of < 100 would be suspicious.

In addition to the provocative tests for open-angle glaucoma just described, there are two tests for narrow-angle glaucoma. Narrow-angle provocative tests should be performed with care because complete closure of the angle, which may occur, often causes rapid and dangerous elevation of intraocular pressure, which requires prompt medical therapy and often emergency surgery. Therefore, these tests should only be done when an ophthalmologist trained to handle such emergencies is present.

Dark Room Test. The *dark room test* is performed by having the patient sit in a dark room for 60 minutes. Physiologic response causes dilatation of the pupil and crowding of the peripheral iris into the anatomic narrow angle. If a large enough portion of the angle becomes blocked to aqueous outflow, the pressure will rise. If the pressure rises 7 to 8 mm Hg, the eye should be considered at risk for an attack of narrow angle glaucoma.

Mydriatic Test. The same response may occur by dilating the pupil with a short-acting mydriatic eyedrop. This is called the *mydriatic test.* The same dangers of rapid rise in intraocular pressure as may occur with the dark room test are inherent in the mydriatic test. Therefore, only one eye should be dilated at a time, and the pupil should be constricted at the end of the test.

Management

The ultimate pathology in glaucoma is atrophy of the optic nerve. Thus, ophthalmoscopy, though less important in evaluating suspicious cases, is extremely important in following the progression of confirmed glaucoma. The earliest changes show narrowing of the small vessels on the temporal surface of the disc. The temporal disc becomes paler. The central cup gradually becomes enlarged and the central vessels deflected nasally. Eventually, the cup becomes so atrophic that the surface of the disc is undermined and the vessels disappear under the overhang and reappear slightly displaced (Fig. 3–5). The lamina cribrosa appears in the depth of the optic cup. The lamina cribrosa is a mesh-like structure that spans the potential hole in the sclera through which the optic nerve passes. As a rule, field defects are proportional to disc cupping. It is unusual to see field changes without disc changes. Consequently, regular ophthalmoscopic evaluation of the disc is an important facet of glaucoma management.

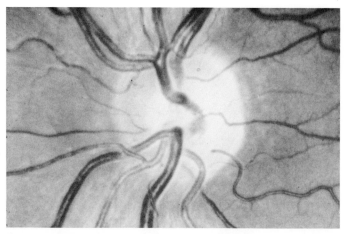

A

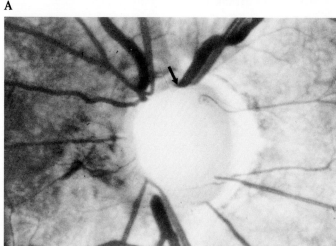

B

Figure 3–5. *A. Normal disc. B. Glaucoma cup. Arrow points to retinal vein as it disappears under overhanging edge of undermined disc. (Photo courtesy of Csaba L. Martonyi, Department of Ophthalmology, The University of Michigan Medical School.)*

TYPES OF GLAUCOMA

A simplified classification of the glaucomas follows:

A. Adult primary glaucomas
  1. Open-angle (chronic simple, simple, or wide angle)

    2. Closed-angle (narrow-angle, angle-closure)
      a. Acute
      b. Chronic
  B. Congenital glaucoma
    1. Primary congenital
    2. Glaucoma associated with congenital anomalies
  C. Secondary glaucoma

Adult Primary Glaucomas

Open-angle or *chronic simple glaucoma* are the most commonly used terms for the type of glaucoma that makes up the majority of glaucoma patients. The pathology lies in reduced aqueous outflow capacity because of narrowing of the trabecular channels.

There are usually no symptoms until vision is lost because of optic atrophy. Examination of the external eye will be normal. Gonioscopy will show normal angle structures. Ophthalmoscopy will demonstrate atrophy of the disc beginning with pallor of the temporal margin and progressing to gradually increasing depth of the optic cup. Visual field defects (Seidel's sign, Bjerrum's scotoma, Rönne's nasal step) will follow the progression of optic atrophy.

This type of glaucoma is the most difficult to diagnose. It usually begins in middle age, and the intraocular pressure becomes elevated gradually. There is a definite hereditary pattern, which should raise the index of suspicion in this group. If the patient is identified early, the major decision is determining the point at which treatment should be initiated. The principle is to begin treatment when the pressure is at a high enough level to cause glaucomatous damage or when damage can be documented by disc or field changes. Most ophthalmologists would agree that pressures in the mid-30s are capable of causing eventual damage. Below that level, treatment is usually withheld unless evidence of disc damage is present.

Medical therapy is the first line of defense in open-angle glaucoma. Control of the pressure in the high teens or low 20s is usually sufficient to prevent progression. This control is sometimes not possible by medical means, and surgery becomes necessary.

THERAPY. Most physicians prefer pilocarpine as the initial therapy. This drug is prepared in drop form in percentages ranging from ¼% to 10%, but there is probably little increase in the effectiveness of concentrations above 4%. It constricts the pupil and causes contraction of the ciliary muscle. These actions open the outflow channels and permit increased aqueous outflow. Treatment is usually begun with pilocarpine 1% or 2% two to four times a day. The strength and frequency are varied on the basis of pressure response.

Some patients, particularly younger patients, cannot tolerate the symptoms of contraction of the ciliary muscle (ciliary spasm). This will change the refractive error i.e., the eye will become more myopic. These patients may be able to adjust if an epinephrine drop is added to the regimen. Epinephrine causes slight dilatation of the pupil. These drops work by reducing aqueous formation and increasing outflow. They are often used in conjunction with pilocarpine, and, in fact, several companies market combinations with various concentrations. The epinephrines often work independently. They are used in 1% or 2% solutions two or three times a day. They have a higher incidence of causing conjunctival irritation than pilocarpine and must be kept refrigerated to maintain their effectiveness.

A newer drug, timolol (Timoptic), has many of the advantages of pilocarpine without the disadvantages of ciliary spasm. It has a longer action and needs to be used only two times a day. Long usage of pilocarpine may lead to some tolerance. The substitution of carbachol for pilocarpine is often recommended when pilocarpine tolerance develops. Carbachol acts much like pilocarpine, and the two can often be interchanged indefinitely as tolerance to the other develops.

Decamarium and phospholine iodide are the other commonly used miotics. They are more potent and longer acting than pilocarpine or carbachol. They have the disadvantage of being more irritating, and they also cause vasodilatation, which may thicken the iris. Thus, these drops are contraindicated for narrow-angle glaucoma. They are often used in aphakic eyes.

When eyedrops are not effective, oral carbonic anhydrase inhibitors often will reduce aqueous production enough to control pressure. Acetazolamide (Diamox) is the most popular of this type of drug. It is used 125 to 250 mg two to four times a day. It also comes in a 500 mg timed release capsule which can be used every 12 hours. The carbonic anhydrase inhibitors can be used in conjunction with glaucoma eyedrops. Unfortunately, they have annoying side effects. Nausea is common. Numbness and tingling of the extremities and a general feeling of malaise are also frequent. In addition, some eyes become resistant to the drug after prolonged use. Therefore, an eye that requires acetazolamide for adequate control may eventually require surgery.

Patients with glaucoma need to have a good emotional support system. They are apprehensive over the potential threat to their sight. The chronicity of their eye disease makes them fearful of blindness. Through education, the public is aware that glaucoma is one of the leading causes of blindness. The nursing staff should have as a prime goal the education of the patient as to the kind of eye health care that is necessary for him.

Nurses should be open and frank with patients. The patients should be aware that the sight that they have lost is gone forever because of damage to the optic nerve. However, it is well to make the patient aware, in a positive manner of what he can do to prevent any further loss of sight, such as instilling eyedrops on time and at the specified intervals. A diagram may be utilized to assist the patient in understanding the condition and the need for medication.

Patients should be aware of the inconvenience that constriction of the pupils may cause. During early morning or at dusk it is more difficult for the patient to see because of pupillary constriction. Normally one's pupils dilate in the dark and constrict in a brightly lighted area. Patients, therefore, must adjust to this inconvenience and plan their lives accordingly. It is more difficult for patients to be in transit in unfamiliar surroundings at this time or to try to read or do other activities that they may be able to manage easier at a different time of day.

When acetazolamide or another carbonic anhydrase inhibitor is given the patient must be cognizant of taking the medication as prescribed. If the patient develops the untoward symptoms of nausea or malaise, with tingling and numbness of the extremities, he must be encouraged to continue the drug. Physicians usually try to switch the drug in hopes that one of the other carbonic anhydrase inhibitors will be better tolerated by the patient. Generally, however, it is found that if patients do not tolerate one carbonic anhydrase inhibitor, they will not tolerate the others. The drug is given to prohibit the formation of aqueous in the ciliary body. It is necessary therefore, for patients to be encouraged and to have positive reinforcement from family and friends of the importance of maintaining therapy while feeling poorly. Patients become distressed at their general feeling of illness and feel that the treatment is worse than the consequences of their disease. Chronic glaucoma progresses very slowly and it might take many years to notice significant visual loss. Therefore, the patient needs to be warned of the "creeping, sneaky thief of sight" that glaucoma can become.

Periodic examinations are essential to adequate glaucoma control. Tonometry should be performed at each visit. Visual fields are an important yardstick of progression. They should be performed at least yearly and more frequently if the intraocular pressure is poorly controlled. The nurse clinician should be familiar with these techniques and be able to perform them when indicated. The clinician can do much to alleviate apprehension and to encourage appropriate medical consultation when it is deemed advisable. (See also Chap. 9, Testing for Glaucoma, p. 256).

Group sessions may prove helpful to some patients. The opportunity to learn that others share similar problems is at times helpful. Also patients can encourage one another to maintain the therapeutic regimen. Patients do find ways of coping that they may share and thus encourage a more discouraged peer.

SURGERY. When visual field changes and optic disc changes progress in spite of maximum medical therapy, surgery must be considered. There are three basic types of surgery for open-angle glaucoma: external filtering procedures, internal filtering procedures, and ciliary body destruction.

There are many types of external filtering procedures. They all have the same purpose, which is to form a drainage channel from the anterior chamber through the sclera just behind the limbus. The aqueous drains under the conjunctiva forming a conjunctival bleb and is then absorbed into the conjunctival blood vessels or slowly migrates through the conjunctiva into the tear fluid.

A large flap of conjunctiva is dissected with its attachments at the limbus. A hole is then made through the sclera into the anterior chamber in the area of the limbus, using a knife incision, enlarged with a scissors, a special punch, or a small trephine. Frequently, cautery is applied to the scleral wound edges. A recent innovation that has gained widespread acceptance makes use of a partial-thickness scleral flap with the entrance into the anterior chamber placed under the scleral flap (trabeculectomy) (Fig. 3–6). The opening through the sclera into the anterior chamber is generally 2 to 4 mm in length. A peripheral iridectomy is then performed by grasping the exposed iris through the opening in the sclera. The iris is tented above the sclera and cut with a

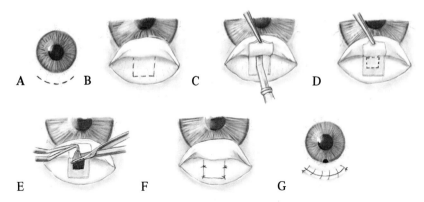

Figure 3–6. *Trabeculectomy. Glaucoma filtering procedure. A. Proposed conjunctival incision. B. Conjunctiva reflected; outline of proposed scleral flap. C. Dissection of scleral flap. D. Outline of proposed partial thickness scleral excision in bed of scleral flap. E. Scleral excision performed; iridectomy being performed. F. Scleral flap closed. G. Conjunctival wound closed; note dark iridectomy.*

scissors. The iridectomy prevents the iris from being pushed against the scleral opening and blocking the outflow. Attempts have been made to incarcerate a wick in the scleral incision to maintain its patency. The most popular technique has been to incarcerate the iris into the wound. This is done by causing the iris to prolapse through the entrance to the wound. The pupil margin is then exposed, and a radial cut is made the full width of the iris. One or both sides of the cut is then incarcerated in the incision and the remainder of the iris replaced into the anterior chamber. This operation is called *iridencleisis* and at one time was very popular, but has been replaced by the newer techniques.

The procedure is completed by carefully resuturing the conjunctiva and tenons to obtain a watertight closure.

The two most important considerations in performing a successful filtering procedure are (1) the proper formation and closure of the conjunctival flap and (2) the proper placement of the scleral opening. If the closure of the conjunctival flap is not watertight, aqueous will leak out from under the bleb, and the anterior chamber will remain flat. This will lead to inflammatory changes, which will often close the scleral opening and eventually scar the conjunctiva resulting in a nonfunctioning bleb. The scleral opening must be placed far enough posterior to avoid tearing the anterior attachment of the conjunctival flap, but far enough anterior to avoid damaging the insertion of the iris and ciliary body.

The so-called internal filtering procedure is better known as *cyclodialysis*. Its purpose is to create a cleft between the anterior chamber and the potential space external to the choroid and ciliary body.

The procedure is performed by opening the conjunctiva and exposing the sclera in one quadrant (usually a superior quadrant) about 4 to 6 mm behind the limbus. A knife is then used to cut through sclera, progressing slowly to guard against damaging the choroid. Most surgeons prefer a circumferential incision about 3 mm long. A spatula is then inserted through the incision and, while pressing the tip against the sclera, the spatula is maneuvered into the anterior chamber in a manner that will produce a cleft about 3 to 5 clock hours in size. The spatula is then removed and the scleral and conjunctival incisions sutured.

The reason this operation works is poorly understood. Probably, the aqueous is absorbed by the outer choroidal surface. This operation is much favored in aphakic eyes because the standard filtering procedures often fail when vitreous clogs the scleral fistula. Cyclodialysis does not usually result in as great a lowering of pressure as can be obtained by filtering procedures.

If all else fails, partial destruction of the ciliary body can be carried out by using applications of diathermy or cryothermy to the ciliary body. These applications are made to the surface of the sclera over the ciliary body and, in the case of cryothermy, may be applied through the conjunctiva and the sclera. The name of the operation is *cyclodiathermy* or *cyclocryothermy*. Effectively, actual scars develop in the ciliary body reducing the aqueous output. More recently a special type of laser has been developed to perform this operation. The laser is applied to the surface of the sclera rather than through the pupil. Its use is limited to the few centers that have this type of laser.

These operations are usually reserved for eyes that have lost useful vision because of uncontrolled glaucoma. They may be temporizing procedures, and they often do not achieve the required result. They can be repeated, but the result is often loss of vision and a phthisical eye. However, occasionally excellent control of intraocular tension and visual improvement does result.

Following all glaucoma operations, cycloplegics and steroid eyedrops should be used until all traces of iritis subside. This is particularly important after filtering procedures, since prolonged iritis might cause the fistula to scar closed or the conjunctival flap to scar against the sclera.

PREOPERATIVE NURSING CARE. Patients are admitted to the hospital the day before surgery. Usually the patient is apprehensive about his forthcoming surgery. Time should be taken to explain hospital procedures as well as operative procedures to aid in allaying some of the patient's apprehension and anxiety. The patients do fear blindness and therefore the positive outcomes of surgery are important to reinforce.

It is important that good glaucoma control be maintained from the moment of admission to the hospital. Since there often is an unavoidable delay in obtaining the proper medication from the hospital pharmacy, the attending physician should be encouraged to instruct his patients to bring their medication with them. This permits uninterrupted treatment.

If patients are being treated with anticholinesterase eyedrops (such as phospholine iodide) and general anesthesia is planned, it is wise to substitute pilocarpine drops for two or three weeks preceding surgery, since low blood pseudocholinesterase activity may interfere with general anesthesia. The anesthesiologist should be informed if a patient has been taking an anticholinesterase drug because use of succinylcholine (Anectine) may cause prolonged apnea. The second problem that may occur after a filtering operation is a severe inflammatory response. This inflammation may result in development of anterior and posterior synechiae, which block the filtration area.

A preoperative medication is ordered. Meperidine (Demerol) may be contraindicated because of its side effect of nausea and vomiting. Frequently, patients with glaucoma cannot tolerate this drug. Morphine sulfate, 8 to 15 mg, and hydroxyzine (Vistaril), 25 to 50 mg, are given intramuscularly an hour before surgery. Flurazepamhydrochloride (Dalmane) 15 or 30 mg can be given at bedtime the evening before and 1½ hours before surgery.

POSTOPERATIVE NURSING CARE. Postoperative nursing care is the same as for any surgical patient. Vital signs of blood pressure, pulse, and respiration should be taken until they are stable.

The patient returns from the operating room with the operated eye patched. The operated eye is usually patched for cleanliness, as there can be bloody serosanguineous drainage.

Miotic eyedrops may be ordered at specific intervals for the unoperated eye. The operated eye may be constricted by use of miotic therapy. Constriction of the pupil aids in preventing closure of the bleb and in maintaining free flow of aqueous. Pilocarpine is frequently the drug of choice and one drop is instilled three or four times a day.

If miotic therapy is instituted, it is continued for approximately four days; then the pupil is dilated with a mydriatic to prevent the formation of posterior synechiae.

In most procedures, miosis is not preferred, and the operated eye is dilated with a mydriatic cycloplegic such as atropine.

Carbonic anhydrase inhibitors are not needed after the filtering operation as the formation of an anterior chamber with free flow of aqueous is usually helpful to maintaining a functional filtering bleb. However, if the unoperated eye demands, carbonic anhydrase inhibitors are continued.

Activity orders are liberal. Most patients are permitted bathroom privileges the day of surgery. Patients generally are told not to lie on the operated side to avoid any risk of pressure on the operated eye.

Pain or discomfort in the operated eye varies. Usually Tylenol gr X or Tylenol No. 3 (two tablets) suffice to relieve the discomfort. Postoperative nausea and vomiting vary with individual patients. An antiemetic is ordered and generally suffices to relieve the discomfort. Meperidine is contraindicated for discomfort since it frequently causes nausea and vomiting. Patients with glaucoma frequently have nausea and vomiting due to increased intraocular pressure.

Tonometry can be performed in the early postoperative period. Therefore, a tonometer should be accessible should the surgeon need to use one. Patients are discharged on the third or fifth postoperative day or at the earliest possible time. It is important for patients to return periodically to their ophthalmologists. Tonometry examinations may be done weekly for a period of time and then monthly. Visual fields are done to determine the progression of loss of vision.

Ideally, medical therapy should not be necessary following surgery. In fact, many patients do require postoperative glaucoma drops or oral therapy or both. If medical therapy is required, its conscientious administration is just as vital as it was before surgery. The nurse can play an important part in explaining the need for continuation and encouragement.

Angle-Closure Glaucoma

Angle-closure glaucoma occurs when the iris bunches up in the periphery of the anterior chamber and prevents access to the angle structures by the aqueous, thereby causing rapid and uncontrollable elevation of the intraocular pressure. The pressure will often soar above 80 mm Hg. The vision is hazy because the cornea becomes edematous. There is marked injection of the conjunctiva, and the pupil is dilated to about 5 to 6 mm and is fixed (does not respond to light). There is extreme eye pain, and often nausea and vomiting. This clinical picture led to the term *acute congestive glaucoma.* It is best to think of it as an acute attack of narrow-angle glaucoma. It is also important to realize that all eyes with congestive glaucoma are not due to narrow-angle attacks, and the treatment will be markedly different if the angle is open.

Narrow-angle glaucoma may exhibit a pattern of transient attacks of lower rises in pressure. The eye does not become congested and the symptoms may be limited to slight blurred vision or halos around lights (both due to minimal corneal edema), headaches, or browaches. These symptoms usually occur in the early evening as it becomes dark and the pupil dilates. This syndrome is called *chronic narrow-angle glaucoma.*

THERAPY. The treatment of narrow-angle glaucoma is surgical. Medical therapy should be used to control the pressure prior to surgery.

Medications. Pilocarpine again is usually effective because it maintains a small pupil and pulls the peripheral iris out of the angle. The strong miotics (e.g., phospholine iodide) should not be used because they cause vascular engorgement and, thus, swelling of the iris. This phenomenon may counteract the effect of the miosis. In acute glaucoma, the iris often becomes paralyzed by the high pressure. The miotics are not effective, and systemic medication must be employed to lower the pressure. Usually, pilocarpine will be effective if the pressure can be reduced. Oral acetazolamide may be effective if the patient is not vomiting. An even more effective medication is an oral solution of glycerine. It comes prepackaged as Osmoglyn 50% in 6 oz bottles and is given at the rate of 1 to 1.5 g/kg of body weight. Unfortunately, this solution may initiate nausea, headache, and vomiting and thus may be poorly tolerated in acute glaucoma because the patient is often already nauseated. It works by increasing the osmolarity of the blood and dehydrating body tissues, including the eye. Other hyperosmolar agents will work the same way, and intravenous mannitol 20% for adults, or 5 to 10% for children, has become the most widely prescribed medication for this condition. It is given at a rate of 1.5 to 2 g/kg of body weight for adults or 1.5 g/kg of body weight for children. Usually a marked drop in intraocular pressure occurs within one-half hour. Intravenous acetazolamide, 250 to 500 mg, can be given in place of, or in conjunction with mannitol or oral glycerine. In severe acute glaucoma, acetazolamide alone is usually not effective, and it rarely is necessary to enhance the mannitol effect.

Surgery. Once the pressure is controlled, surgery should be performed. The definitive procedure is a peripheral iridectomy. This is effective because an opening between the anterior and posterior chamber is made just in front of the chamber angle, which allows passage of aqueous from the posterior chamber into the anterior chamber and allows the aqueous to reach the angle and its outflow structures in one area. This breaks the cycle, causes the peripheral iris to flatten, and allows fluid to reach the angle 360°.

The operation can be performed under a conjunctival flap at the limbus or through the clear cornea. The incision is made parallel to the limbus and about 3 to 4 mm in length. If the limbal approach is used, slight pressure on the globe will usually cause the iris to prolapse through the incision. It can be grasped with a forceps, a small piece excised, and the iris massaged back into the anterior chamber, thereby avoiding entering the anterior chamber with an instrument. If the corneal approach is used, the forceps must be inserted into the anterior chamber. The iris is then tented through the incision, and the remainder of the operation is the same. After the iris is returned to the anterior chamber, the pupil should be constricted with pilocarpine. If the pupil becomes round and small, one can be rather certain that no iris is incarcerated in the wound. The incision is then closed with a fine suture.

The pupil should be dilated and steroids begun on the first postoperative day and continued until all iritis has ceased. Persistent iritis will cause adhesions between the lens and the iris, effectively close the iridectomy, and negate the effect of the surgery.

There is a high incidence of an acute narrow-angle glaucoma attack occurring in the other eye within a few years of the initial attack. Thus, most ophthalmologists will recommend miotic therapy for the fellow eye. If the anterior chamber angle is very narrow, prophylactic peripheral iridectomy should be advised.

If the glaucoma was due purely to closed angle, treatment should not be necessary after the eye becomes quiet. In some cases of chronic narrow-angle glaucoma, trabecular incompetence may be superimposed on narrow-angle glaucoma. If so, the pressure will remain elevated after a successful peripheral iridectomy, and medical therapy should be started in the same fashion as would be initiated for simple glaucoma. If medical therapy does not control the pressure, a filtering procedure can be performed.

Primary Congenital Glaucoma

Primary congenital glaucoma is a recessive hereditary disease. It is more common in males, and about two-thirds of the patients have bilateral disease. Most cases are present at birth and almost all of the remainder are discovered by the third year. This type of glaucoma occurs because the two mesodermal layers, which normally split beginning about the fifth fetal month, fail to separate completely and leave a thin membrane of iris stroma over the angle structures. This membrane prevents the aqueous from reaching the outflow channels.

Typical symptoms are photophobia, tearing, and blepharospasm. The cornea is hazy, often becoming opaque, and it eventually becomes enlarged. The eye enlarges because of increased pressure on elastic tissue. This results in stretching of the cornea and breaks in Descemet's membrane. The corneal edema is mostly due to the breaks in Descemet's membrane with the elevated intraocular pressure forming a pressure gradient pushing fluid into the cornea. If the condition is diagnosed early, there is a good chance that vision can be saved. However, if the corneal edema persists, the cornea may become opaque, and the prognosis for functional vision is poor. Disc cupping may occur early, but is probably more reversible than in adults. Tonometry is sometimes misleading because of the flattened cornea and the elasticity of the tissues; and general anesthesia, if light, will cause a decrease in intraocular pressure occasionally as much as 50 percent. Thus, a high index of suspicion should be maintained in any child with persistent unexplained photophobia, tearing, or both.

THERAPY. Medical treatment is generally ineffective, and the results of filtering procedures have been disappointing. Goniotomy is the surgical procedure of choice. The operation is performed by inserting a fine knife, which has the appearance of a miniature harpoon, through the cornea just anterior to the limbus. While observing the angle with a special gonioscope lens, the point is carried across the anterior chamber, and the abnormal tissue is cut by sweeping the knife across as large an arc of the angle as possible, exposing the underlying angle structures. If bleeding occurs, it is important to turn the head away from the side of the eye that was operated so that angle structures are not blocked (i.e., if the nasal side of the left eye is treated, turn the head on the left side.

Tension is normalized in about 40 to 50 percent of eyes with one operation. This procedure can be performed multiple times. Some series show that normalization is achieved in 80 percent or more of treated eyes if multiple operations (as many as four or five) are performed.

Glaucoma Associated with Congenital Anomalies

The term *congenital glaucoma* is generally restricted to primary congenital glaucoma, in which incomplete angle cleavage occurs in fetal life. However, there are several other congenital anomalies that carry a high incidence of glaucoma. In these others, the glaucoma is rarely present at birth and may not occur until middle age. These glaucomas are variously classified as secondary, congenital, infantile, and juvenile.

The following touches on some of the more common conditions. Sturge-Weber Syndrome (hemangioma of the face, nevus flammeus) is the commonly seen (usually unilateral) port-wine stain (Fig. 3–7). Glaucoma develops on only the side of the face involved by the hemangioma. The mechanism of the glaucoma is poorly understood, and treatment is often ineffective. Filtering operations are complicated by the frequent presence of vessels on the iris and in the angle. Aniridia is a congenital anomaly. Some rudimentary iris tissue is present at the iris root. This tissue usually becomes adherent to the already abnormal angle. The prognosis, even with surgery, is poor. Neurofibromatosis (Recklinghausen's disease) may be associated with glaucoma if it involves the upper eyelid. Iris nodules are often present and may have some relationship to the glaucoma. Angle structures, however, are poorly developed. Persons with microcornea usually will experience acute angle-closure attacks but often not before the second or

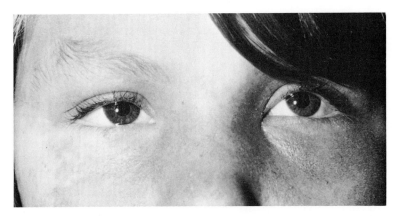

Figure 3–7. *Port-wine stain surrounding left eye across the nose and be-low right eye. (Photo courtesy of Frank Flanagin, Associated Retinal Consultants, Detroit.)*

third decade. Clinically, the diagnosis and treatment are the same as for adult angle-closure glaucoma.

Secondary Glaucoma

The secondary glaucomas constitute roughly 30 percent of all glaucoma. By definition, the etiology is an ocular disease other than a developmental abnormality. There are many possible causes, and the prognosis and treatment are as varied as the causes.

Inflammation may cause elevation of pressure in several ways. Active iritis or cyclitis may cause increased aqueous outflow above what the outflow channels can handle. Treatment is usually medical, but may be complicated because miotics, which normally would increase outflow capacity, will increase the inflammation. Steroids, which may calm the iritis, often aggravate the glaucoma. Therapy must be tailored to reflect these various responses. Often carbonic anhydrase inhibitors will be necessary to reduce the pressure while using cycloplegics (atropine) to control the iritis. Topical steroids often do not contribute to the elevated pressure and can be added to the regimen. In other cases, topical steroids are not tolerated but systemic steroids are.

Iritis may cause glaucoma in several other ways. The cellular debris may clog outflow channels. In the acute phase this is treated with cycloplegics (atropine). After the iritis is controlled, miotics may be necessary to counteract permanent outflow damage. The inflammation may cause adhesions of the peripheral iris to the cornea or to angle structures. These adhesions in the anterior chamber are called *synechiae* and when found in the chamber angle are called *peripheral anterior synechiae.* They may occur in narrow bands or may completely obliterate the angle over its 360° circumference. If 25 percent of the angle is open and normal, ocular tension will probably remain normal.

If the angle is totally occluded by peripheral anterior synechiae, filtering surgery will be necessary. Synechiae may cause adherence of the pupil to the lens or vitreous. If these posterior synechiae completely seal the pupil, aqueous will be unable to reach the anterior chamber and build up behind the iris, and the iris will bulge forward. The condition is called *iris bombé* and can be relieved by a peripheral iridectomy.

Any debris in the anterior chamber can block outflow channels. Lens remnants, following lens capsule rupture, or hemorrhage. or tumor cells are all capable of blocking the trabecular meshwork. Often these pressure rises are transient, and normal control returns as soon as the underlying pathology is controlled. Temporary miotic therapy is often sufficient, but, if it fails, carbonic anhydrase inhibitors are usually effective.

Mechanical blockage of the angle may develop secondary to (1) swelling of a lens as it becomes cataractous, (2) dislocation of the lens into the anterior chamber, or (3) dislocation of the lens into the pupil. These conditions will lead to an acute angle-closure attack. Medical control of the condition should be attempted, because it is safer to operate on a quiet normotensive eye. Often intravenous mannitol is necessary to break the cycle and restore normal pressure. Surgical removal of the lens will be necessary.

Trauma, meaning a direct blow to the eye, will often cause hemorrhage in the anterior chamber because of rupture of an iris blood vessel. The iris root may be torn from its attachment to the sclera and a cleft may be seen gonioscopically. This finding will confirm the existence of previous trauma. The cleft is not the cause of the glaucoma and the exact cause is not well understood. Glaucoma may develop immediately or years later. Treatment should follow the same pattern as in simple glaucoma. Surgery should be reserved for those eyes uncontrolled medically.

Thus, in all types of secondary glaucoma, the underlying cause should be corrected first. Any residual elevated pressure should be controlled in the same fashion as chronic simple glaucoma if the angle is open and treated as narrow-angle glaucoma if the angle is closed.

DISEASES OF THE IRIS

INFLAMMATIONS

The iris is an integral part of the uvea and as such will be involved
to a greater or lesser degree with inflammations of the choroid
and ciliary body. (See Chap. 7, Retinal Inflammation, p. 159.)
Certain diseases have a predilection for the choroid, and others
tend to involve the iris primarily.

Diagnosis

Symptoms may be as innocuous as slightly blurred vision and mild
irritation, or may be severe enough to cause incapacitation because
of pain. The diagnosis is confirmed by demonstrating the presence
of cells in the anterior chamber. Slit-lamp examination using a
narrow slit of light will show these cells very clearly (just as
particulate matter can be seen in the beam of swimming pool
lights). These cells often deposit in clumps on the posterior surface
of the cornea or on the anterior surface of the lens. Deposits on
the posterior cornea are called *keratic precipitates* (KP). KP are
easily seen with the slit lamp but often are large enough to be
seen with the naked eye. They will absorb when the iritis is controlled. If massive cellular response occurs the cells may settle
inferiorly in the chamber angle and form a level. This is called
a hypopyon.

In all but the mildest cases, there will be engorgement of the
scleral vessels surrounding the corneal limbus. This can be distinguished from conjunctival injection by its localization to a band
around the limbus. This injection is so typical that a term, *ciliary
flush,* has been coined to describe this phenomenon. Even in the
presence of conjunctival injection, the ciliary flush can be recognized as a purplish discoloration along the limbus. Blurred vision
is caused by debris in the anterior chamber, by cellular deposits
on the posterior corneal surface, and by spasm of the ciliary
muscle secondary to associated inflammation in the ciliary body.
Ciliary spasm will cause an accommodative-like response in the
lens and will blur distance vision. Because the iris is inflamed
there will be irritation when the musculature contracts, so that
pain on exposure to light is common and becomes worse as the
iritis becomes more severe. It is easy to understand this because the
same response occurs in an irritated skeletal muscle.

The cause may be obvious if local pathology is present. Trauma to the cornea will usually cause some iritis, and, if corneal ulceration develops, the iritis may be prolonged. Bacterial, viral, or fungal involvement of the cornea is usually accompanied by an iritis. Herpes simplex and herpes zoster are relatively common causes of iritis. It is often difficult to evaluate the anterior chamber for signs of iritis because of corneal edema or ulceration. If this much disruption of the cornea is present, iritis should be presumed to exist.

Hypermature cataract changes may lead to an autoimmune reaction resulting in iritis. This condition should be suspected any time iritis is discovered in the presence of a mature cataract. Treatment requires complete cataract removal.

There are many systemic diseases that demonstrate iritis. Mild to moderate iritis may occur with the acute infectious diseases of childhood, such as mumps, varicella, rubeola, and rubella. Foci of infection have been implicated. Therefore a search for occult infections, such as sinusitis, abscessed teeth, or pelvic inflammatory disease is indicated. Rheumatoid arthritis and its variants—gout, Reiter's syndrome, and psoriasis—all have a high incidence of iritis.

If an obvious local cause is not present, a complete history and general physical examination should be performed, with special attention given to foci of infection. Routine blood and urine tests, including complete blood count, differential, and a serum multiphasic screen, with attention to the rheumatoid factors, should be obtained. It is important that a thorough initial evaluation is carried out because anterior uveitis may become chronic, and long-term, continuous, or intermittent therapy may be necessary.

Treatment

Treatment is nonspecific unless a definite cause has been determined. Even in such cases, cycloplegics are used to set the iris at rest by relieving light sensitivity, and topical steroids are used to reduce inflammation. Antibiotics are unnecessary unless the iritis is associated with a corneal ulcer. Systemic steroids occasionally are necessary. Rapid pain relief is often achieved by the use of cycloplegics without analgesics. Thus, a rapid-acting cycloplegic should be instilled as soon as the diagnosis is made. In addition, dilatation of the pupil prevents adhesions (posterior synechiae) from binding the pupil to the surface of the lens and preventing dilatation at a later date.

Occasionally, elevated intraocular pressure may be present. This is usually due to blockage of outflow channels by debris and cells from the anterior chamber. It must be distinguished from acute glaucoma. Acute glaucoma is characterized by a slightly dilated pupil which does not react to light, hazy cornea, and absence of circumcorneal flush. Iritis, on the other hand, even in the presence of elevated pressure, shows a small pupil and a clear cornea.

The irritated eye may result from a mild condition or a serious problem that threatens vision. Proper diagnosis and early treatment may save the eye (Table 3–1).

Table 3–1. *Similarities and Dissimilarities of Conjunctivitis, Iritis, and Acute Glaucoma. Differential Diagnosis of the Red Eye.*

Physical Assessment (signs and symptoms)	Conjunctivitis	Iritis	Acute Glaucoma
Eye pain	No	Variable	Yes
Conjunctival injection	Yes	Mild	Yes
Circumcorneal flush	No	Yes	Variable
Conjunctival secretion	Yes	No	No
State of cornea	Clear	Clear	Hazy
Light sensitivity	Mild/variable	Intense	Variable

Nursing Care

In nursing care of iritis, the most important aspect is to maintain dilatation of the pupil, thereby preventing posterior synechiae from forming. A mydriatic cycloplegic type drug such as atropine 1% drops given several times a day is generally instituted to maintain mydriasis. Topical steroids are usually used in conjunction with the cycloplegic. Occasionally systemic steroids will be given, along with or in place of the topical steroids.

Since secondary glaucoma is a complication, it is important to take tonometry measurements frequently and to watch for symptoms of glaucoma.

There frequently is eye pain, which will vary from mild discomfort to extreme pain. This is usually relieved as soon as the cycloplegics take effect but analgesics or narcotics are sometimes necessary. Compresses may be soothing and can be used as needed.

TRAUMA

Blunt Trauma

Trauma does not usually affect the iris unless there is a direct injury to the eye. Blunt trauma may cause dilatation of the pupil, disinsertion of the base of the iris, radial tears at the pupil margin, circumferential tears along the iris base (iridodialysis), and hemorrhage.

Traumatic mydriasis will occur immediately upon the receipt of a direct blow to the eye. Usually the pupil will return to normal within seconds and function normally thereafter. However, if the blow is severe enough the mydriasis may remain for days to weeks and in some cases become permanent. The mechanism of the injury is not well understood and there is no effective treatment.

Occasionally a blow is serious enough that the iris is torn away from its attachment to the sclera. This rarely occurs over more than three clock hours. The presence of such pathology indicates severe anterior chamber trauma, and there is a high incidence of glaucoma in these eyes. The glaucoma may develop years after the injury. Instead of tearing the base of the iris from the sclera, the iris itself may tear in a circumferential direction just anterior to its attachment to the sclera. This is called an *iridodialysis* (Fig. 3–8). If the iridodialysis is large enough, the pupil may become eccentric (off center). This usually does not affect vision and no treatment is necessary, although surgical repair can be carried out by suturing the peripheral iris back into position using a suture through the sclera.

Radial tears at the pupil margin cause an irregular pupil and occasionally reduced pupillary reaction, but otherwise do not affect function.

Penetrating Wounds

Penetrating wounds of the eye may disrupt the iris, but the major concern is the damage done to the other ocular structures. Occasionally, if the iris is severely damaged, an attempt to reposition or fashion a better functional or cosmetic iris will be attempted

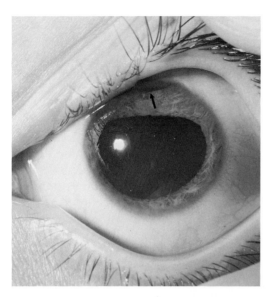

Figure 3–8. *Irregular pupil. Arrow points to iridodi-*
alysis. (Photo courtesy of Csaba L. Martonyi,
Department of Ophthalmology, The University
of Michigan Medical School.)

as part of the repair of corneal or lens damage. One important
point should be made: frequently, a small foreign body may enter
the eye and cause very little discomfort. It may even enter just
peripheral to the corneal limbus and have its entrance wound
hidden in edematous conjunctiva. The presence of a small unexplained hole in the iris is definite proof that something has pene-
trated the eye. Careful ophthalmologic evaluation, including an
x-ray of the orbit, is indicated.

TUMORS

Malignant tumors of the iris are uncommon. The most common
tumor is the *nevus.* Most nevi appear as localized pigmented areas
of flat or slightly denser iris tissue. The eye should be photo-
graphed or diagrammed and observed at prolonged (yearly) intervals. The patient should be advised that this lesion could undergo
malignant change and should be encouraged to report any change
in size or color. If a question exists, fluorescein angiography
can be performed. (See Chap. 7, Photography, p. 154.) A nevus
should show no hyperfluorescence.

Malignant Melanoma

Malignant melanoma appears as an elevated lesion and will show hyperfluorescence. Melanomas of the iris are very benign when compared to choroidal melanomas and there is no need for haste in making a diagnosis. (See Chap. 7, Tumors, p. 192.) In most instances these tumors can be excised, even if they extend into the ciliary body, and the results and survival rates are excellent.

Metastasis to the iris is rare. The reason is that the blood supply to the iris is limited. Most of the tumors arise from breast and lung. The treatment should be directed at the primary tumor. However, if complications develop, excision or radiation of the metastatic lesion may be necessary.

HETEROCHROMIA

A comment should be made about the iris color. There is a wide variation in iris color, but normally a person has the same color iris in each eye. *Heterochromia* is the term used for a difference in iris color. This condition may be congenital but more often it is secondary to intraocular disease. Retained iron (either from a foreign body or massive hemorrhage) in the eye will eventually cause the iris to take on a rusty color. A nevus or melanoma may be large enough to cover most of the iris. Chronic iritis may give a muddy brownish color. There is a specific type of chronic iritis called *heterochromic iritis,* which causes the affected eye to be paler than the other. Therefore, a high index of suspicion should be carried when seeing heterochromia.

DISORDERS OF THE IRIS

Under most circumstances, the pupils of both eyes are equal and react equally to light and accommodation. Unequal pupils may signal traumatic mydriasis or sluggishness secondary to chronic iritis or synechiae. They may also signal systemic disease.

HORNER'S SYNDROME

Another notable example of unequal pupils occurs in Horner's syndrome (miosis, anhidrosis, and slight ptosis). This syndrome results from disruption of the cervical sympathetic nerves on the same side as the findings. It is important to recognize this syndrome since it is frequently caused by serious systemic diseases (e.g., multiple sclerosis, thyroid tumors, metastatic tumors, mediastinal tumors, lesions of the apex of the lung, occlusion of the posterior inferior cerebellar artery, tumors of the cervical cord, among others).

ARGYLL ROBERTSON PUPIL

The Argyll Robertson pupil is a miotic pupil; it reacts to accommodation but not to light. It is seen most commonly in late stages of neurosyphilis, and is helpful in alerting the examiner to this diagnosis.

SURGERY

Surgical intervention in disease of the iris is uncommon. Most iris surgery is done as a part of cataract or glaucoma surgery. The most common procedure is the iridectomy. When the iris is cut it does not repair itself and a permanent defect remains. Thus, iridectomy will provide an auxiliary opening to insure adequate aqueous flow into the anterior chamber. The anterior chamber is entered within 1 mm of the limbus. The iris is picked up with a fine forceps and cut with a small scissors.

Plastic repair for iris trauma is rarely needed, but can be done by using fine (10–0) polyester sutures. The size of the corneal incision will depend upon the exposure needed. Removal of an iris tumor will require a larger corneal incision than an iridectomy for a glaucoma procedure. The corneal incision is closed with sutures.

ANTERIOR CHAMBER

Inspection of the external eye should always include evaluation of the depth of the anterior chamber. This is important for two reasons. If the chamber is shallow, instillation of dilating drops may initiate an attack of acute narrow-angle glaucoma. Second, the presence of a shallow anterior chamber following injury may alert the examiner to a perforating injury. It is not difficult to learn to evaluate anterior chamber depth. Since the vast majority of eyes have normal chamber depth, merely looking at each eye critically will soon allow one to develop a sense for the normal. Directing a flashlight from the side will allow this estimation to be made more easily. If there is a question, slit-lamp examination

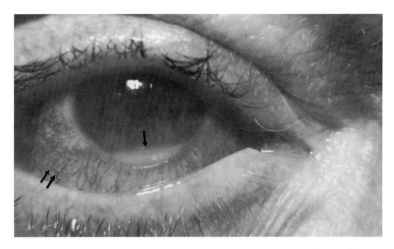

Figure 3–9. *Single arrow shows hypopyon. Double arrow shows conjunctival and episcleral injection. (Photo courtesy of Frank Flanagin, Associated Retinal Consultants, Detroit.)*

will usually provide the answer. If not gonioscopy must be performed.

In the presence of severe iritis or endophthalmitis from any cause (or very rarely in the presence of an intraocular tumor, especially retinoblastoma) so many cells may fill the anterior chamber that they will settle inferiorly and form a whitish yellow crescent. The term used to describe this is *hypopyon* (Fig. 3–9). Its importance is that it signifies intense reaction in the anterior chamber. It will clear as the primary condition resolves.

A diagnosis may sometimes be facilitated by draining some of the aqueous and studying the fluid by serum chemistry techniques and the cells by cytology. Drainage of the anterior chamber is called *paracentesis.* It is done by inserting a small knife or a sharp needle through the cornea just anterior to the limbus.

Trauma may cause hemorrhage to develop in the anterior chamber due to rupture of the iris vessels. Usually only a small amount occurs and the cells can be seen floating in the aqueous only by slit-lamp biomicroscopy. Occasionally so much bleeding will occur that it will settle inferiorly and form a level. This condition is called a *hyphema.* Hyphemas usually will absorb within several days but if the entire chamber fills, the outflow channels may be blocked by the debris and the blood may fill the entire anterior chamber and form a dark clot. This has been called an *8-ball hemorrhage* and is an ominous sign. It is not uncommon for an initial mild hemorrhage to begin to absorb and two to five days after injury a second larger hemorrhage will occur.

Treatment of hyphema requires bed rest for about five days. After five days it is unusual for a secondary hemorrhage to occur. If the intraocular pressure remains normal, no further treatment is usually necessary. Some ophthalmologists feel miotics will cause more rapid absorption of blood; others feel cycloplegics will paralyze the iris movement and lessen the chance of rehemorrhage from weakened iris blood vessels. Good statistical evidence is not available to solve this dilemma.

The best method of obtaining complete rest is to patch both eyes and keep the patient on bed rest. Elevating the head of the bed will encourage settling of the blood in the anterior chamber and may prevent synechiae formation. One must be on constant alert for the development of elevated intraocular pressure, which may rise above 50 mm Hg. Acetazolamide may control the pressure but repeated hemorrhaging will often render all medical therapy ineffective. There is usually pain at the moment of recurrent hemorrhage, and pain may linger if the pressure becomes elevated. Patients with eye pain often feel very lethargic—a warning sign of recurrent anterior chamber hemorrhage or pain secondary to elevated intraocular pressure associated with hyphema in a child.

If the hemorrhage and intraocular pressure cannot be controlled medically, particularly in the presence of an 8-ball hemorrhage, which is not absorbing, surgical intervention is necessary. Paracentesis, often with irrigation of the anterior chamber using fibrinolysin to dissolve the clot, may be helpful. However, the need for surgical intervention, is, itself, a poor prognostic sign.

SELECTED READINGS

BOOKS

Allen, H. *May's Diseases of the Eye* (24th ed.). Baltimore: Williams & Wilkins, 1968.

Duke-Elder, S. (Ed.). *System of Ophthalmology.* Vol. III. *Cornea and Sclera:* Pt. I. *Diseases of the Outer Eye,* Pt. II. *Conjunctiva.* Vol. IX. *Diseases of the Uveal Tract.* Vol. X. *Diseases of the Retina.* Vol. XI. *Diseases of the Lens and Vitreous; Glaucoma and Hypotony.* Vol. XIII. *The Ocular Adnexa Lids, Lacrimal Apparatus, Orbit and Para-orbital Structures.* St. Louis: Mosby, 1969.

Sugar, H. S.   *The Glaucomas* (2nd ed.). New York: Hoeber Med. Div., Harper & Row, 1957.

ARTICLES

Blodi, F. C.   Glaucoma. *American Journal of Nursing* 63(3): 78-83, 1963.
Durkee, D., and Bryant, B. G.   Drug therapy reviews—Drug therapy of Glaucoma. *American Journal of Hospital Pharmacy* 35: 682-690, 1978.
Soll, D. B.   Glaucoma. *Nursing Digest,* 3: 9, 1975.

CHAPTER 4 ⸻

MUSCLES OF THE EYE

ANATOMY

The movement of each eye is controlled by six muscles (Fig. 4–1).
All are flat ribbon-like muscles that attach to the eyeball by flat
tendons about 10 mm wide. Four of the muscles originate at the
posterior aspect of the orbit, run straight forward, and insert
into the sclera about 6 to 8 mm behind the limbus. These are the
medial rectus (MR), lateral rectus (LR), superior rectus (SR), and
inferior rectus (IR) muscles. They are called the recti. The two
other muscles are called oblique (O) because of the direction of
their insertion into the sclera. The superior oblique (SO) muscle
arises from the posterior orbit slightly medial to the origin of the
superior rectus; it passes forward to the trochlea, a U-shaped
fibrocartilaginous structure that attaches to the roof of the orbit
a few millimeters behind the superior orbital rim at the supraorbital notch (a depression you can feel on yourself about one-
third of the distance temporal from the nose along the superior
orbital rim). The superior oblique muscle becomes a tendon just
behind the trochlea, runs through the trochlea and bends back
at an angle of about 50° to insert into the sclera behind the insertion and under the belly of the superior rectus muscle. The
inferior oblique (IO) muscle arises several millimeters behind the
inferior orbital rim and directly below the supraorbital notch.
It extends posteriorly and temporally at an angle of 50° to the
line of sight. It courses between the inferior rectus muscle and the
inferior orbital wall and inserts behind the insertion and under
the belly of the lateral rectus muscle.

Nerve supply to all the eye muscles occurs through the cranial
nerves. Divisions of the third cranial (oculomotor) nerve supply
the medial, inferior, and superior rectus muscles and the inferior
oblique muscle. The fourth cranial (trochlear) nerve supplies the
superior oblique muscle, and the sixth cranial (abducens) nerve
supplies the lateral rectus muscle. The nuclei of the third and
fourth cranial nerves lie in the midbrain while that of the sixth
lies in the pons, and the nerves course through the intracranial

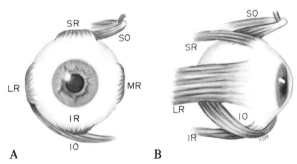

Figure 4–1. *Extraocular muscles. A. Anterior view. B. Lateral view.*

cavity under the brain to reach the posterior aspect of the orbit, where they enter the orbit and supply the muscles.

MUSCLE ACTION

Contraction of a muscle turns the eye toward that muscle (Fig. 4–2). For example, contraction of the right lateral rectus turns the right eye toward the right. The horizontal muscles, the medial and lateral rectus, turn the eye to the right or left. The four remaining muscles, the vertical muscles, elevate or depress the eye. The oblique muscles have their greatest effect when the eye is turned nasally and the vertical recti when the eye is turned temporally. For example, when the eye is turned toward the nose, the superior oblique turns the eye down and the inferior oblique, up. When the eye is turned temporally, the superior rectus turns the eye up and the inferior rectus, down. One can envision this if he remembers the direction the muscles take in inserting on the sclera and remembers that the muscles exert their effect by contraction.

It is obvious that each muscle does not work independently of the others. When any muscle is contracting, its antagonist (muscle), the one that produces the opposite effect, must be relaxing. In fact, for any eye movement, even for looking straight ahead, all six muscles are constantly working to maintain smooth movement or steady fixation.

In addition, the two eyes must work together if they are to maintain constant focus. The muscles that produce movement of each eye in the same direction are called *yoke muscles* (Table

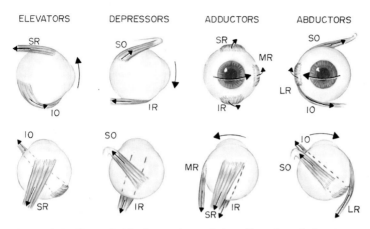

Figure 4–2. *The individual muscles and the effect that their contraction has on eye rotation.*

Table 4–1. *Yoke Muscles and Antagonists*

Antagonists	Yoke Muscles
Medial rectus–Lateral rectus	Right medial rectus–Left lateral rectus
Superior rectus–Inferior rectus	Right lateral rectus–Left medial rectus
Superior oblique–Inferior oblique	Right superior rectus–Left inferior oblique
	Right inferior rectus–Left superior oblique
	Right superior oblique–Left inferior rectus
	Right inferior oblique–Left superior rectus

4–1). That is, one muscle is the yoke muscle of the other. Thus, if the right eye looks up and in (inferior oblique contracting), the left eye must look up and out (superior rectus contracting), and the movement must be smooth and equal in each eye. There are six major positions to which the eyes must be able to move. These six positions test the primary function of the muscles of each eye and are called the cardinal positions of gaze (Table 4–2, Fig. 4–3).

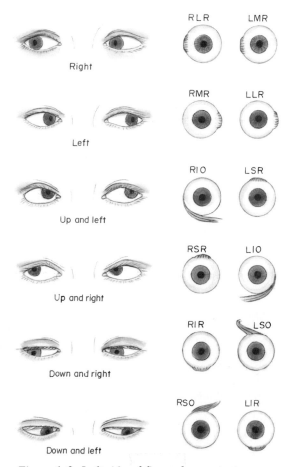

Figure 4-3. *Left side of figure demonstrates eye position. Right side of figure demonstrates muscles contracting to produce that eye rotation.*

Table 4-2. *Six Cardinal Positions of Gaze*

Direction of Gaze	Muscles Involved
Right	Right lateral rectus–Left medial rectus
Left	Right medial rectus–Left lateral rectus
Up and right	Right superior rectus–Left inferior oblique
Up and left	Left superior rectus–Right inferior oblique
Down and right	Right inferior rectus–Left superior oblique
Down and left	Left inferior rectus–Right superior oblique

STRABISMUS

Strabismus is the pathologic condition in which only one eye is directed at the intended object of regard. Functionally, this results in *diplopia,* commonly called *double vision.* There are two basic classifications of strabismus: paralytic and nonparalytic.

Paralytic, or paretic (the term more frequently used) as its name indicates, occurs because of pathology that weakens the pulling power of the muscle. Paresis may occur because of damage to the nucleus (of the nerve), to the nerve or the muscle itself.

Nonparalytic, or nonparetic, strabismus results from a poorly understood abnormality in the fusion ability of the two eyes without paralysis of a muscle. This malfunction is poorly understood.

Nonparetic strabismus is classified into (1) accommodative, (2) nonaccommodative, and (3) combined accommodative-nonaccommodative.

Accommodation is the function that allows a person to vary the focus of the lens. In addition, there is a reflex action that turns both eyes in as the accommodation increases power to focus at near vision. If a person is emmetropic, the focusing mechanism is completely relaxed at distance, and the turning in reflex usually coordinates well with the amount of focusing. If a person is hyperopic (i.e., farsighted), it is necessary to actively focus the eyes just to maintain clear distance vision. Occasionally, the hyperopic person cannot learn to coordinate this abnormal focusing-turning in relationship, and the eyes turn in either constantly or possibly only at near. If a person is myopic (nearsighted), the eyes are focused at near when the accommodation is relaxed. Thus, the myopic person needs less accommodation than normal, and his eyes may turn out.

The abnormal accommodative element can be neutralized by prescribing the proper optical correction to relax the eyes' focusing mechanism when viewing a distant object. Thus the eyes will function like emmetropic eyes and the accommodative reflex can function normally. The nonaccommodative element can then be dealt with by other means.

MEASUREMENT OF DEVIATION

To plan treatment of strabismus, and to evaluate progress, the amount of the deviation must be measured. Many tests have been devised to obtain these measurements. Most of these tests use

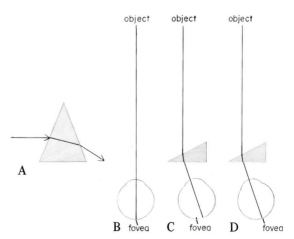

Figure 4–4. *A. Path of light through a prism. B. Normal progression of a central light ray to the fovea. C. A light ray deflected by a prism off the fovea. D. The eye rotated to focus a deflected light ray on the fovea. (If the eye is directed, as in strabismus, the appropriate prism will deflect a straight light ray onto the fovea.)*

prisms, and the amount of the deviation is designated by the amount of prism necessary to neutralize it.

Prisms

A prism works by changing the direction of the light rays as they go through it. Light rays are bent toward the base of a prism. Thus, when a prism is placed in front of the eye, the eye will perceive an image coming from a new direction, deflected toward the apex of the prism (Fig. 4–4).

When one eye is deviated, prism may be added in front of the eye until the image of the object of regard appears to be coming from the direction of the deviation. This will be the angle of the deviation or the angle of the strabismus.

The unit of measurement is the prism diopter. It is defined as the amount of prism necessary to deviate a beam of light 1 cm at 1 meter from the prism.

The most commonly used test for the angle of deviation is called the prism cover test. The test is performed in the following manner. The patient is asked to fix on an object and one eye is covered.

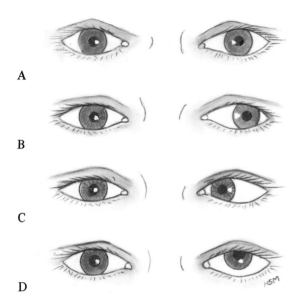

A

B

C

D

Figure 4–5. *Eye positions while fixing a light. A.
Straight eyes. (Note light reflexes just nasal to the
center of the pupil in each eye.) B. Left exotropia.
C. Left esotropia. D. Left hypertropia.*

The cover is then transferred directly to the opposite eye, and the
amount and direction of the movement to take up fixation by the
eye which had been under the cover, is noted. An appropriate
size prism is then placed over the fixing eye. The eye will move
into a new position, since it will appear that the object is coming
from a new direction. The cover is then moved back over the
original eye, and again the movement of the eye is observed.
Prism power is added or subtracted until the eyes do not move
to take up fixation as the cover is moved back and forth over
each eye.

As soon as one begins to think about measuring muscle abnormalities it will become obvious that there are several basic
groups: eyes deviated inward, eyes deviated outward, and so on
(Figs. 4–5, 4–6). These groups have special names derived from
the position of the deviating eye: *exo* out, *eso* in, *hyper* up.
(*Hypo* is not used. Since a vertical deviation always has a hyper
eye, the deviation is called hyper and the elevated eye is named,
for example, right hyper.)

In addition, as soon as one begins to do cover tests, he will

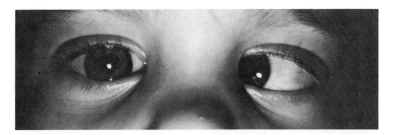

Figure 4-6. *Esotropia, left eye. (Note light reflex. Child is fixing light.)* *(Photo courtesy of Frank Flanagin, Associated Retinal Consultants, Detroit.)*

discover that many patients who do not have strabismus show movement when the cover is moved back and forth over the eyes. These people have a latent deviation, which they are able to control when both eyes are uncovered, but this deviation becomes evident when the fusion mechanisms relax in the absence of a need to fuse (prevent diplopia). This latent deviation is termed *phoria.* The manifest deviation or strabismus is termed *tropia.* Thus, we name deviation by combining the direction, size (in prism diopters), and latency, for example, a 24-diopter (prism diopter) exotropia or a 12-diopter esophoria, or perhaps a combination horizontal and vertical strabismus, a 20-diopter exotropia with a 6-diopter right hypertropia.

Light Fixation

Several other methods of evaluating strabismus are helpful, particularly as screening devices. The easiest and most commonly used test involves having the patient fix on a light. The examiner then observes the light reflex in the patient's pupils. The reflex normally falls about 1 mm nasal to the center of the pupil in each eye. If the reflex falls to the temporal side of the normal position, the eye is turned in and the patient has an esotropia and if the reflex falls to the nasal side, the patient has an exotropia. Occasionally the deviation may be so small that it is difficult to identify by observation alone. The examiner may then cover one eye while watching the uncovered eye. If the uncovered eye does not move, it was fixing before the cover was applied. The cover is then removed and after a moment placed over the other eye, and again the uncovered eye is observed. If the second eye does not move, it may be assumed that no strabismus is present. This test will also demonstrate phorias. The examiner must watch the eye that has been under the cover as the cover is being removed. If a phoria is present, he will see movement of the eye to resume fixation.

MADDOX ROD TEST. There is a subjective test that can be used to demonstrate phorias and tropias. It makes use of a rippled glass called a *Maddox rod.* If a light is used as a fixation point and the Maddox rod is held over the eye, the light appears as a line. The line is perpendicular to the ripples in the glass. By directing the line successively in a horizontal and vertical direction, vertical or horizontal phorias or tropias can be demonstrated. Measurement can be performed by using prisms.

TREATMENT

There are three basic methods of treatment for strabismus: (1) prisms, (2) orthoptics, and (3) surgery. These methods apply only after the full optical correction has been prescribed.

Prisms

Prisms, although extremely useful in measuring deviations, are much less helpful in treatment. When they are used they are mounted in glass frames. Frequently, the deviation is so large that the prisms would be cosmetically unacceptable, or the deviation changes with different positions of gaze, making the prisms useless. Prisms are most helpful for small vertical deviations.

Orthoptic Techniques

Orthoptics is an important method of treatment; orthoptic instruments are used to teach the patient to fuse. Orthoptics involves exercises to help train the patient in using the eyes together. These exercises often may be done at home but several instruments are important in teaching the patient to recognize normal visual relationships.

EYEPATCHES. The most common orthoptic device is the occlusive eyepatch. Patching is necessary when the vision in one eye drops because that eye has crossed. When an eye crosses, the binocular effect results in double vision. If this occurs in a child, he soon learns to overcome the double vision by disregarding the image from one eye, thus re-establishing single vision. However, when he does this, he suppresses the vision in the crossing eye. If this suppression occurs for a long enough time, the vision in the eye becomes permanently suppressed and the condition is called *amblyopia ex anopsia* (amblyopia of disuse). The primary method of treatment is to patch the better seeing eye continuously and force the patient to use the poorer seeing eye. The most rapid improvement occurs if the patch is not removed, except to change it.

Most of you are familiar with the beige, adhesive backed patch, which is the most common type of occlusive patch. This patch rarely limits a child's activities and patched children may be seen everywhere. Patching often must be continued for a year or more before the vision improves to normal levels and in some instances the vision never returns to normal. Patching is usually stopped when no improvement is seen after six months of adequate patching. The ideal result is return of vision equal to the better seeing eye.

VISUAL TRAINING. Importance of the need for return of vision lies in the fact that re-establishment of binocular vision depends on having the vision close to equal in the two eyes. Once this has been achieved, the eyes must be aligned so that the patient can use them together. At this point, orthoptic techniques may be employed by the orthoptic technician in an attempt to train the control centers to reassert coordinated binocular movements. The most useful technique for this purpose employs the use of an instrument called an *amblyoscope* (Figs. 4–7, 4–8). It employs two small projectors so that a separate image may be presented to each eye. Each picture is mounted on a movable arm. In this way, the arms may be moved into the crossing position of the eyes, and the patient will perceive the images projected as a person with straight eyes would see them. Usually, images in each projector will be slightly different; for example, one image might be a house with a chimney and without a door and the other, the house with a door but without a chimney. If the patient sees a house with something missing the technician knows that he is suppressing one eye. However, if the patient sees a house with a chimney and a door, the technician knows that he is using both eyes, and exercises can proceed to move the eyes into normal position by changing the position of the arms of the amblyoscope while maintaining the total picture (a house with a chimney and a

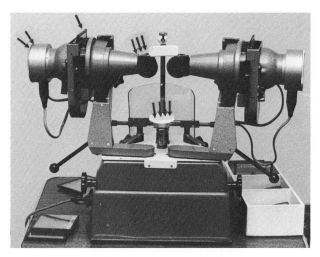

Figure 4-7. *Amblyoscope viewed from patient's side. Single arrow shows slide. Double arrow shows light source. Triple arrow shows eye piece. Quadruple arrow shows chin rest. (Photo courtesy of Frank Flanagin, Associated Retinal Consultants, Detroit.)*

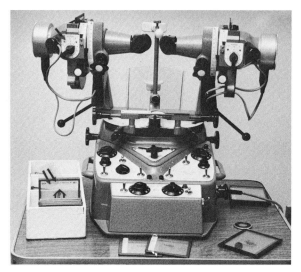

Figure 4-8. *Amblyoscope. Viewed from operator's side. Single arrow shows rheostat to control intensity light source. Double arrow shows slide box with a slide of house without chimney. (Note that dual controls allow all functions to be adjusted separately for each eye.) (Photo courtesy of Frank Flanagin, Associated Retinal Consultants, Detroit.)*

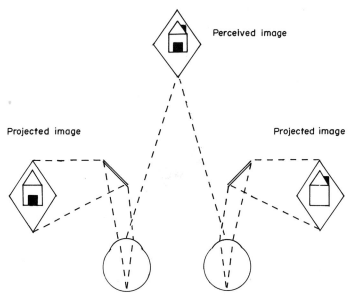

Figure 4-9. *Concept of the amblyoscope. A separate image is projected into each eye. If the patient's fusion ability is normal, he will perceive the completed picture.*

door) in focus (Fig. 4-9). If the eyes can be moved into the normal position on the amblyoscope, other exercise techniques can be carried out at home. These exercises must be practiced daily, aiming to maintain normal eye position without the instrument. If this is successful, normal binocular vision may be achieved.

It is apparent that these types of exercises require a great deal of patient cooperation. Unfortunately, strabismus usually occurs when a child is too young to cooperate satisfactorily and by the time he is old enough to cooperate the habits are so ingrained that orthoptics is much less effective. Surgery, therefore, is usually necessary. Even when surgery is needed, orthoptics is almost always necessary if binocular vision is to be achieved. This takes the form of patching and amblyoscope training to develop binocular appreciation before surgery, and exercises after surgery to train binocular function.

Surgery

There are two basic types of eye muscle operations, the recession and the resection. Each can be used on any muscle, and multiple

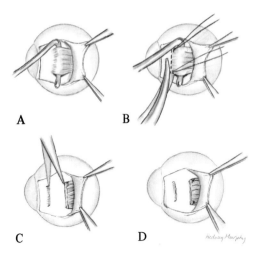

Figure 4-10. *A. Conjunctival incision demonstrating muscle hook underneath horizontal
rectus muscle. B. Suture placed through
either edge of muscle just behind the insertion. Dotted line indicates the proposed
scissors cut. C. Muscle resutured to sclera at
the measured distance illustrated by caliper.
D. Procedure complete, ready for resuturing
conjunctiva.*

muscles are often operated either at the same operation or at
separate operations to achieve the desired result. The name of
the operation literally describes what is done. First an incision
must be made in the conjunctiva and the muscle isolated. If a recession is to be performed, sutures are placed at the edge of the
muscle just behind its insertion in the sclera (Fig. 4-10). The
needles are left on the suture. The muscle attachment to the
sclera is then cut and the muscle allowed to retract. A measuring
caliper is used to mark the exact amount of recession desired.
A small mark is placed on the sclera, and the muscle is resutured
to this spot using the previously placed sutures.

If a resection is to be done, the approach to the muscle is the
same. The amount of muscle to be resected is marked with the
calipers and either sutures are placed at this spot or a muscle
clamp is placed across the muscle, as the surgeon prefers. The
muscle is then cut anterior to the sutures or clamp and then the
anterior part is cut away from its insertion (Fig. 4-11). The cut

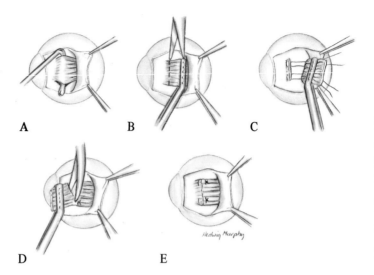

Figure 4–11. *A. Conjunctival incision demonstrating muscle hook underneath horizontal rectus muscle. B. Muscle clamp applied to muscle just anterior to the proposed resection line. Dotted line indicates the line where the muscle will be severed from its insertion. C. Sutures placed through the original insertion and through the muscle just behind the muscle clamp. D. Sutures have been tied. Excess muscle is trimmed. E. Shortened muscle resutured to the original insertion. Conjunctiva ready for closure.*

end of the muscle is then sutured to the original insertion, shortening the muscle.

Recessions weaken muscles. Resections strengthen muscles. There are certain anatomical and functional limits to how much a muscle may be recessed or resected. Horizontal muscles are usually recessed 5 mm or less and resected 8 mm or less. Vertical muscles usually are recessed or resected 5 mm or less.

The "maximum" surgery on a muscle usually changes the position of the eye about 15 prism diopters. Thus, the amount of surgery is varied depending on the amount of deviation. For example, a right esotropia of 30 prism diopters might be treated by recessing the right medial rectus 5 mm (weakening) and resecting the right lateral rectus 8 mm (strengthening the antagonist). If the esotropia were nonparalytic, some surgeons would prefer to do a bilateral medial recession, which would weaken the turning in power of each eye. In this example even though only the right eye turns in, the surgical effect is on the relationship between the two eyes and would have a net effect of straightening the right eye. If the deviation were less than 15 prism diopters, the surgeon might elect to operate on only one muscle or he might split the amount of surgery by doing less than the maximum surgery. For example, in the case of 15° esotropia, he might elect to do 3 mm recessions of each medial rectus muscle.

The primary goal of all muscle surgery and orthoptic training is restitution of binocular vision. Care must be taken surgically, so that an acceptable cosmetic result will develop if binocular vision does not develop. Postoperatively, it is not uncommon for the eyes to drift out of alignment over a period of years if the patient does not maintain binocular vision. Further surgery may be necessary if this occurs.

PREOPERATIVE NURSING CARE. Most surgery is done on children, and therefore, we have made particular reference to them.

Preoperative explanation should be in terms the child understands. This preparation should begin in the doctor's office when the time for surgery is decided upon.

Children are usually in the hospital for a short time, one to two days. Some surgeons are now doing this surgery in surgical outpatient departments; hence, the child arrives at the hospital the morning of the procedure and returns home that evening. In this way, the child never leaves his own bed or is separated from his family and familiar surroundings.

In giving nursing care the age of the child is important. After the age of 9 months children are aware of their mother's absence, and consequently hospitalization is frightening. Separation causes the child to cry and show signs of separation grief. The child at this age is able to remember, or has a memory. Children of this age group benefit from having a primary care nurse. They respond favorably to a continued relationship with one person.

The 2- to 3-year old fears losing the mother. These years are important as they are the toilet training years. The separation may be regarded as punishment and therefore the hospitalization is accompanied with a sense of guilt.

The child of 4 to 5 years who is hospitalized may exhibit many nervous mechanisms. The child's fears or anxieties may be displayed through nail biting or nail picking, picking at nose, twisting hair around a finger, or other nervous habits. Children of 4 to 5 do fear accidents or death. They frequently will regress to bed-wetting and begin having nightmares. Children of this age have strong attractions to the parent of the opposite sex. The hospitalization to them may represent punishment for their fantasies.

All of these age groups would benefit from a constant relationship. Primary nursing would be a benefit to all of these children, as their primary nurse would be with them when they were undergoing treatments or experiences that are new to them.

Routine blood work and general physical examination can be done before hospitalization. The child usually has been under the physician's care for some time, and these procedures will be less stressful on an outpatient basis.

General anesthesia is usually used, since the surgery is done mainly on young children between one and six years of age. The child may be admitted to the hospital on the morning of surgery or the day before depending on the physician and hospital policy. If surgery is performed in the surgical outpatient department, then no hospitalization is required.

All children, hospitalized and nonhospitalized, receive nothing by mouth from the midnight previous to the morning of surgery. Preoperative medication varies from no medication, a sedative, or combination narcotic and anticholinergic drug.

If a preoperative injection is given, the dosage is in accordance with the child's (age-height-weight) body surface. An example of this would be an anticholinergic such as atropine in combination with a narcotic such as morphine. Some doctors give a barbiturate such as phenobarital sodium (Luminal) or a sedative such as secobarbital (Seconal). These drugs, if used, are given to relax the patient and thereby to relieve some anxiety during the induction phase of anesthesia. Also the anticholinergic decreases secretions and makes intubation easier. Some doctors use an antibiotic eyedrop to remove as many pathogens from the conjunctiva as possible.

General preoperative care for the adult is similar to that given any surgical patient. Adults are frequently admitted the day before surgery. Routine laboratory work is done. They take nothing by mouth from midnight the day of surgery.

Preoperative medications vary with the individual surgeon. Frequently a narcotic, a sedative, and a narcotic potentiator or tranquilizer are given. Therefore meperidine (Demerol) 75 mg and hydroxyzine (Vistaril) 50 mg may be given intramuscularly one hour preoperatively. Atropine is given intramuscularly to reduce secretions and to aid in the induction phase of anesthesia if a general anesthetic is to be given. Pentobarbital sodium (Nembutal) 100 mg is given intramuscularly 1½ hours preoperatively.

POSTOPERATIVE NURSING CARE. On returning from the recovery room, the child should receive general surgical nursing care. Vital signs (blood pressure, pulse, and respiration) should be taken as indicated. The child may or may not be wearing an eyepatch. If patched, the operated eye should be observed for drainage. There is usually no discharge or a minimal amount of discharge. The conjunctiva appears reddened and remains so for approximately one to two weeks. A steroid or antibiotic eyedrop is used three times a day for a week to relieve inflammation. Some surgeons prefer an ointment, since this is soothing and the fundus does not need to be examined (ointments leave a film over the cornea and make funduscopic examination more difficult.) Warm compresses are used by some surgeons three times a day for a week to aid in relieving irritation. These compresses also aid in cleaning the eye if a discharge is present.

The child does suffer from visual disability, so nursing care should be geared to this problem. Postoperative patching of the affected eye is again the individual surgeon's preference. Duration of patching varies from a week, to 24 hours, to no patching. There is little to minimal drainage postoperatively. However, the eyepatch protects the patient from light irritation, whether natural or artificial.

Many children have had unilateral patching as preoperative treatment so they do not find a patch limiting. They can move around their hospital environment with little difficulty. Usual safety precautions initiated for visual disabilities on young children are necessary—for example, during getting in and out of bed, keeping side rails up (be that child or adult), and assisting with meals. In a children's ward, added precautions should be taken against leaving toys on the floor out of (eyepatched) gaze, or range of vision.

A nursery school or kindergarten child may return within two days after surgery. Some surgeons may prefer a week from school, to allow an office visit first. Generally, children do well and are back to their regular routine within several days of surgery.

Postoperative nursing care for the adult is the same as for any surgical patient. Vital signs of blood pressure, pulse, and respiration should be taken every 15 minutes until stable and then once every shift for 24 hours.

Patients return from the operating room with the operated eye patched, for cleanliness and comfort. There may be a slight amount of serosanguineous drainage on the eyepatch. However, frequently there is no discharge present.

Activity orders are liberal, the patient being permitted out of bed and to the bathroom the evening of surgery. Diet is returned to "regular" when the patient is able to tolerate a full meal. Generally, patients do not have nausea or vomiting and are able to eat an evening meal or to begin a regular diet the first postoperative day.

Patients instill a steroid-antibiotic type drop (such as Maxitrol) three or four times a day to lessen inflammation and prevent infection. Discharge is usually the first postoperative day, and the patient goes home with the steroid-antibiotic drop. Eyepatches are given to patients, to avoid the annoyance of natural or artificial light, which by evening can cause reddening, burning, and possibly tearing (epiphora). The patient should be warned of this possibility so that he is not unduly alarmed. Some patients continue to have diplopia, and they should be warned that this may occur. Diplopia may subside as the eyes adjust to their new postoperative situation. Patients may read, watch television, and have normal activity. Frequently they do not return to work for one week. Patients generally return to see their physician within one week of discharge. Generally by this time activity is back to normal.

SELECTED READINGS

BOOKS

Dunlap, E. A. (Ed.) *Gordon's Medical Management of Ocular Disease.* (2d ed.). Hagerstown, MD: Harper & Row, 1976.
Vaughan, D., and Asbury, T. *General Ophthalmology.* (8th ed.). Los Altos, CA: Lange, 1977.

ARTICLE

Hiles, D. A. Strabismus. *American Journal of Nursing* 74(6): 1082–1089, 1974.

CHAPTER 5 —————————

THE LENS

The lens is the most important part of the focusing mechanism of the eye. It contributes about one-quarter of the focusing power of the eye, most of the remainder being developed at the surface of the cornea. However, the lens performs the very important function of accommodation, the ability to change the focus of the eye. The lens is also the site of cataract formation, the most common cause of reduced vision. Cataract is the condition in which the lens becomes partly or completely opaque.

The lens has the appearance of a biconvex glass lens (Fig. 5-1). Its diameter is about 8 mm, and its thickness varies, depending on the state of accommodation, but is approximately 5 mm. It lies between the iris and the vitreous body in close contact with the iris on its anterior surface, and centered in its position by multiple fine fibers called *zonules,* which extend from the ciliary body to the equator of the lens. These zonules attach to the equator of the lens 360° around it and run in a radial fashion to their connections in the ciliary body at the level of the ciliary processes. It is the changes in the musculature of the ciliary body which tent or relax the zonules and, therefore, affect the focus of the lens by changing the curvature of its anterior and posterior surfaces.

ANATOMY

The lens is made up of three major portions:

1. A tough outer clear capsule that completely surrounds it
2. A single row of epithelial cells that lie directly inside the capsule in the anterior portion of the lens only
3. Lens substance

The capsule is secreted by the epithelial cells, and the epithelial cells in the equatorial region form the lens fibers, which continue to be formed throughout life. The lens substance itself can be divided into two general areas, the cortex and the nucleus. The

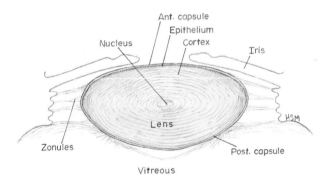

Figure 5–1. *Cross section of lens structure.*

epithelium is constantly forming new lens fibers, and these fibers are the cortex. The anterior and posterior cortices surround a much harder and denser area, the nucleus, which is made up of older lens fibers that have become dehydrated and compressed by the more recently formed lens fibers at the periphery of the lens.

CHEMISTRY

The chemistry of the normal lens is very complex, but its major function is the maintenance of a relatively low water content. Normal body cells concentrate potassium and excrete sodium. Since water tends to move with sodium, any interference with this mechanism causes increased water content in the cell. In the human being, the lens capsule appears to be the site of sodium-potassium transport control, and it has been shown that any injury to the lens capsule will result in increased sodium and water retention in the lens.

The transparency of the lens depends upon its remaining in a relatively dehydrated state. The only pathologic changes that can occur in the lens are variation in water content and opacification of the lens fibers. The changes seen in the chemical concentration of a cataractous lens are related to the disruption of the sodium, potassium, and water balance mechanism. Thus there is an increase in water content, sodium, and calcium, and a decrease in potassium and protein, resulting in opacification.

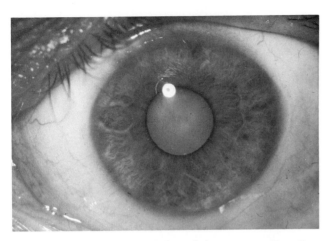

Figure 5–2. *Cataract. Note light reflex on upper edge of pupil. (Photo courtesy of Frank Flanagin, Associated Retinal Consultants, Detroit.)*

CATARACTS

Any opacification within the lens is called a cataract, regardless of its location (Fig. 5–2). Most cataracts occur as gradual senile change and the impetus for development is poorly understood. Some diseases are associated with high incidence of cataract (e.g., diabetes). Congenital cataracts are commonly associated with certain diseases (e.g., rubella). The other common cause is trauma. If the lens capsule is torn, as by a penetrating foreign body, or even damaged by severe blunt trauma of the surface of the eye, a cataract will develop.

SYMPTOMS

What symptoms do cataracts produce? By and large, the only symptom is painless progressive loss of vision. In the so-called senile cataract, the type that develops gradually with age, there is a slow process, often occurring over many years. It is amazing, however, that many people develop advanced cataract changes in one eye without noticing the gradual loss of vision. Only when something causes them to shield the better eye, such as soap in the eye, do they notice the visual loss, and they then describe it as a sudden loss. Other symptoms, such as glare, which is common in a bright light, do occur but are much less important than the major symptom of visual loss. Pain occurs only if the cataract causes (1) marked swelling of the lens, which upsets the normal flow of aqueous, causing acute glaucoma, or (2) rarely, an iritis due to toxins, released by the lens.

INDICATIONS FOR SURGERY

The indication for cataract removal is decrease in vision to a degree that the patient cannot perform normal activities. Thus, a wide variability in visual acuity will justify cataract surgery. For example, a draftsman might be totally unable to perform his work with 20/50 visual acuity, whereas a 70-year-old retiree, who does little else than gardening and watching television, might be very happy with 20/200 visual acuity. The decision as to when to remove a cataract is based on the visual needs of the patient unless other medical or ophthalmic considerations supervene.

Clinically, a cataract is evaluated by its appearance under microscopic examination using the slit-lamp biomicroscope. In addition, the ophthalmoscope is used to confirm that the opacity of the cataract actually interferes with the observation of the retina and progression of light rays through the lens to the retina.

SURGICAL TECHNIQUES

There are two basic techniques for cataract removal: intracapsular and extracapsular. Extracapsular surgery was the primary method used in all patients 40 years ago. As instrumentation improved, it became possible, in most instances, to remove a lens with an intact capsule—that is, intracapsular. Intracapsular removal has become the standard technique. In the last few years, however, new interest has arisen in the extracapsular technique because of the development of a new instrument called the phacoemulsifier.

The advantages of the extracapsular technique center around being able to use a small incision. This technique has been the method of choice for youngsters because once the anterior capsule is opened, the cortical material can be washed out of the remaining capsule and, with a needle and syringe, sucked out of the anterior chamber. However, when the lens ages, the new lens fibers compress the older fibers into a hard nucleus. By middle age, this nucleus is too firm to be broken up and sucked out by a

needle, and if left in the eye will cause a great deal of inflammation. Therefore, a large incision is necessary to remove the nucleus
and, as long as a large incision is to be made, a quieter postoperative eye results by removing the lens within the capsule. Thus,
the intracapsular technique has become the technique of choice by
almost all ophthalmic surgeons.

The introduction of the phacoemulsifier now presents the
surgeon with a choice of technique. The phacoemulsifier uses
ultrasound waves to fragment the hard nucleus, after which the
material can be sucked out of the anterior chamber just as the
cortical material is removed. The advantage is that the phacoemulsifier can be inserted into the anterior chamber through a
3 mm incision as opposed to the 15 to 18 mm incision required
for the standard intracapsular operation.

Because the phacoemulsifier procedure is a new operation,
further experience will be necessary to determine its place in the
handling of cataracts. It challenges a standard procedure that
produces excellent visual results in over 95% of operations performed, but it excites ophthalmologists because of the obvious
advantage of a significantly smaller incision, which would allow
more rapid return to normal activities.

A procedure gaining in popularity is insertion of an intraocular
lens implant following cataract extraction. There are basically
two classifications of intraocular lens implants, the anterior chamber lens and the iris plane lens. The anterior chamber lens fits
snugly into the anterior chamber angle while the iris plane lens has
loops attached to the iris. These loops are made of metal or plastic
and allow the lens to be supported by the iris by having the loops
straddle the iris through the pupil.

The type of lens used depends for the most part on the surgeon's
preference. However, certain iris abnormalities may prevent the
use of the iris plane lens, and some conditions of the eye may
prevent the use of either type of lens.

Cataract surgery can be performed using general anesthesia,
but the large majority of operations are performed under local
anesthesia. Local anesthesia is obtained by placing the tip of a
needle behind the eyeball in the pyramid formed by the four
rectus muscles—in what is called the *muscle cone.* Several milliliters
of anesthetic solution, such as lidocaine (Xylocaine), are then injected. This injection completely anesthetizes the eye and stops eye
movements by paralyzing the eye muscles and markedly reduces
the vision by acting on the optic nerve. In addition, an injection

is made around the lids to paralyze the lids and prevent squeezing during the operation. Local anesthetic is not usually used if the procedure is performed under general anesthesia.

SURGICAL APPROACH

The standard cataract surgery is begun by making an incision in the conjunctiva from about 9 to 3 o'clock (Fig. 5–3). This incision is made about 4 mm behind the corneal scleral juncture (the limbus) and dissected down toward the limbus, a *limbus-based conjunctival flap,* or the incision is started at the limbus and dissected away from the limbus, a *fornix-based flap.*

The purpose is to expose the limbus, where the incision into the anterior chamber will be made. The initial entrance is made with a knife. Most surgeons now use a special type of delicate scissors to enlarge the incision along the limbus from about 9:30 to 2:30 o'clock. Sutures can be inserted before the incision is completed, after it is completed but before the cataract is removed, or after the cataract is removed.

The iridectomy is usually performed at this time. A piece of iris is removed to facilitate aqueous flow from behind the iris, where it is formed, into the anterior chamber, where its outflow channels lie. When the cataract is removed, the vitreous often moves forward and fills the pupil like a plug, stopping the normal flow of aqueous into the anterior chamber, and glaucoma will occur. By making a small hole in the iris at the periphery, there is less chance that the aqueous flow will be blocked. These small holes are called *peripheral iridectomies,* and some surgeons perform two or three as an added safety factor. If the cataract removal appears to be difficult, it is often necessary to perform a complete iridectomy. This involves removing a wedge of iris from the pupil to the periphery of the iris.

At this point some surgeons inject an enzyme, alpha chymotrypsin (Chymar), which decreases the strength of the zonules holding the lens. It is injected behind the iris and usually irrigated out of the anterior chamber after two or three minutes.

The lens is grasped with a suction device known as an *erysiphake,* a capsule forceps, or a cryosurgical probe, and removed from the anterior chamber. If preplaced sutures have been used, they are tied. If not, sutures are now inserted. The number of sutures depends upon the length of the incision, the accuracy of the initial sutures, and the philosophy of the surgeon. The tendency in the

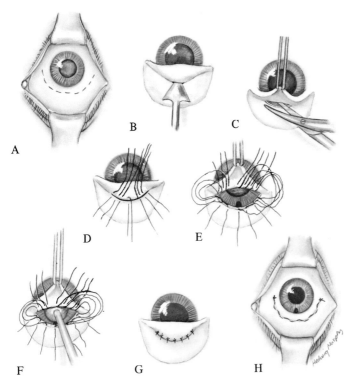

Figure 5–3. *Intracapsular cataract extraction (diagram is aligned
as the surgeon would view the eye—sitting behind patient's head).
A. Planned conjunctival incision (dotted line). B. Conjunctival
flap folded over cornea. Keratome knife is being inserted into the
anterior chamber. C. Scissors enlarging corneal scleral incision.
D. Sutures preplaced before removal of cataract. E. Sutures are
drawn aside giving unobstructed view of anterior chamber.
Note that iridectomy has been made at the 12 o'clock position
(6 o'clock in the drawing). F. Forceps holds incision open while
cryoprobe is placed on surface of cataract and the cataract withdrawn from the eye. G. Corneoscleral sutures tied. H. Conjunctiva
sutured.*

last ten years has been to use more sutures. In the early 1960s,
the average number of sutures was probably three. Ten years
later, the average had increased to five to seven. The increase was
aided by development of finer instruments, needles, and suture
material and by greater reliance on the operating microscope.

The operation is completed by suturing the conjunctival incision.

The phacoemulsification procedure is initiated by making a 3 mm incision through the cornea at the 12 o'clock limbus. A fine hook-like knife (cystotome) is then inserted into the anterior chamber and used to cut and tear a large piece of the anterior lens capsule from 6 o'clock toward 12 o'clock. The capsule is pulled through the incision and excised.

The cystotome is then used to lift the nucleus out of the lens capsule into the anterior chamber. The phacoemulsifier instrument is inserted in the anterior chamber. The ultrasound waves break up the nucleus, and the suction mechanism removes the debris. After the nucleus has been removed the suction apparatus is placed into the capsular pocket and sucks out the remaining lens cortex.

A peripheral iridectomy can then be performed through the small corneal incision. The incision is closed with a single suture and the procedure is completed.

An intraocular lens can be introduced after an intracapsular, extracapsular, or phacoemulsification operation. However, an incision of at least 120° is necessary to insert the lens safely. Therefore, if phacoemulsification is used, the incision must be enlarged before lens insertion. It is important that the inner surface of the cornea is not scraped by either the lens or the instrument holding the lens. Many surgeons fix the iris plane lenses with a fine (10–0) suture placed into the iris. Precise wound closure is essential, since a flat anterior chamber will create contact between the cornea and lens. All of these maneuvers require the ability to see with sharp detail. Therefore, most authorities agree that intraocular lens implantation should be performed only under microscopic control.

The visual results obtained with an intraocular lens are superior to any other type of postcataract lens system. However, the surgical and postsurgical complication rate seems to be slightly higher than with the standard procedure, and the long-term results have not yet been seen.

Most surgeons feel that at the present time intraocular lenses should be reserved for those patients over 65 years of age.

If a complication occurs during surgery, it is recommended that an intraocular lens not be used.

Extracapsular cataract extraction in youngsters can be performed by inserting a large (18 to 22 gauge) needle through a small corneal incision into the lens. The lens cortex can then be sucked out of the capsule since no nucleus is present. An alternative is to tear the anterior capsule (as was described under phacoemulsification) and then suck out the cortex.

Whenever the capsule is left in the eye, it may become opaque after months or years. This is called a *secondary cataract* or *secondary membrane.* It is treated by inserting a narrow knife through the cornea and cutting through the membrane into the vitreous. This technique usually opens a clear window and allows clear vision again. If this is unsuccessful, the membrane may be removed with vitrectomy techniques (see Chap. 6), or the eye must be opened, as with a standard cataract operation, and the membrane removed with forceps, cryoprobe, or scissors.

Hospital Procedure

PATIENT ORIENTATION. Preoperative nursing care should begin with the explanation by the surgeon and his office team of the prospective hospitalization. Upon admission to the hospital, the patient should be oriented to his immediate surroundings, and hospital routines such as meal time, evening snacks, if available, and so on.

Since patients who are admitted to the hospital for cataract extraction are usually in the older age group and have decreased vision in one and possibly both eyes, safety precautions are important. These patients may not be familiar with hospital surroundings, and therefore walking any distance may result in a possible fall. The patient's vision is decreased, blurred, and lacking in depth perception. Hence, elevations in the floor such as ramps may cause the patient to lose his balance. Because this lack of depth perception can cause patients to fall and injure themselves, many patients utilize a walking cane outdoors or in unfamiliar surroundings indoors to prevent them from stumbling or falling on rough, uneven sidewalks, curbings of various heights, and elevations or depressions on flooring, such as change in the depth of carpet pile.

In the case of various height curbs, the walking cane can be lowered to the street before the patient steps off the curb. This then is a warning to him of the approximate height of the curb and the size step he will be taking. The same premise holds true for walking up or down stairs. The walking cane can be placed on the step preceding the patient's footstep. This procedure assists him in knowing the height of the step as well as when the last step has been reached.

Since the hospital furniture is unfamiliar to the patient, he may have difficulty judging the distance before sitting. Patients should be told not to sit until they feel the chair behind their legs. Also they should reach for the arm of the chair, if it is an armchair, to stabilize their balance when changing from standing to sitting.

While many institutions discourage walking around the hospital, they do permit walking to the dining room or to a patients' lounge. Accidents such as falls can occur even when steps and unusual elevations are not present in the immediate physical structure. Therefore, it is wise to walk initially with the patient to the dining room or the lounge, to familiarize him with these areas.

Individual hospital policy will dictate the use of side rails as well as height of the adjustable beds. Some institutions have a rigid policy and others are more lenient, letting the nurse assigned to the patient judge his ability to get in and out of bed.

WORKUP. Patients should have routine laboratory work, ECGs, and chest x-ray if necessary. Some surgeons choose to have an internist evaluate the patient preoperatively, usually on an outpatient basis.

PREPARATION OF THE EYE. Most surgeons use an antibiotic drop or ointment for several days or a week preoperatively. The night before surgery the patient is given a sedative to rest well. On the morning of surgery, an antibiotic eyedrop is instilled to lessen the pathogens in the conjunctiva. A "dilating series" consisting of a cycloplegic drug and, if desired, a mydriatic, is used preoperatively to dilate the pupil. Most surgeons give a sedative 1½ hours before surgery. An injection of a narcotic and, if desired, a cholinergic blocking agent is given one hour preoperatively to lessen the patient's apprehension and to make local anesthesia more tolerable. A frequently used preoperative medication is one and a half grain 100 mg of secobarbital (Seconal) as the sedative and 25 mg promethazine hydrochloride (Phenergan) and 50 mg of meperidine (Demerol) for the narcotic potentiator and the narcotic.

POSTOPERATIVE NURSING CARE. After the operation, the patient's activity depends on the number of sutures used to close the wound. Generally all patients having cataract extractions are permitted some degree of bathroom privileges, which may or may not be allowed immediately after surgery but are usually permitted the evening of the day of surgery. Some surgeons permit the patient to be ambulatory on the first postoperative day. Patients are reminded to move slowly and carefully for at least three to four weeks to avoid straining.

Upon going home, patients are encouraged to be careful and to avoid falling. Reading and light activities are permitted immediately. Heavy work should not be undertaken for 4 to 12 weeks after surgery.

Since the use of the phacoemulsifier includes a very small incision (approximately 3 mm), the postoperative limitation of activities for these patients is considerably less than with the other surgical techniques. Many patients return to normal activities within several days.

Complications. The greater the number of sutures to close the corneoscleral wound, the less danger of distortion of the wound by patient activity. The patient is told not to lie on the operated side, to avoid putting pressure on the eye. Pressure on the globe, squeezing the eye, or straining may increase intraocular pressure and may separate the wound sufficiently to cause loss of the anterior chamber. Loss of the anterior chamber may not be dangerous, however, because the wound may reapproximate, and newly produced aqueous will re-form the anterior chamber. However, there is a danger that the iris might become incarcerated in the wound or prolapse through the wound and distort the pupil. In an inflamed eye, the iris may be drawn into the anterior chamber angle, often leading to glaucoma.

Another danger is vitreous loss—prolapse of vitreous through the wound. This is the most serious complication of cataract surgery other than intraocular infection because it may cause vitreous hemorrhage or retinal holes. Retinal holes often lead to retinal detachment.

Intraocular infection is the most dreaded complication of intraocular surgery. Measures taken to prevent this complication are antibiotic eyedrops preoperatively; also, before closure, an injection of gentamycin sulfate (Garamycin) or some other broad-spectrum antibiotic is frequently used.

Operating rooms do have strict policies to prevent such infections. A primary concern in operating rooms is airborne infection. The masks worn by all operating room personnel should cover nose and mouth. They should be changed every hour since masks at best do not give much protection when talking, laughing, or coughing. Operating room scrub suits should not be worn to and from any other area of the hospital unless the surgeon returns to change suits before rescrubbing. All shoes should be reserved for operating room use. Most operating rooms do require non-conductive booties to be worn over the shoes.

Air circulation, air conditioning, and filtering are all major concerns in maintaining an environment that would prohibit operative infections.

The use of single-dose medications and saline is preferable. Air to be injected should also be sterile.

The treatment of endophthalmitis, should it occur, consists of massive doses of antibiotics systemically, intracameral (into anterior chamber), intravitreal (into vitreous), and subconjunctival injections. Intraocular cultures may be taken and culture and sensitivities determined to begin appropriate therapy.

Patching. Eyepatching varies with the individual surgeon's preference. Some keep the eye patched for six days to lessen the danger of squeezing or squinting due to irritation from natural or artificial light. On the other hand, some patients feel quite comfortable with a patch and wear it for several weeks (Fig. 5–4). Other surgeons feel an eyepatch is unnecessary and simply tape the inside of a rigid metal or plastic shield to provide a closed environment, to keep the eye clean while protecting it from trauma.

For four to eight weeks, the patient uses a rigid metal or plastic shield taped securely over the eye during sleep, to prevent the unconscious rubbing or bumping of the eye (Fig. 5–5). The shield can be removed during the day, and the patient is permitted to wear his or her own glasses as a protection against bumping or rubbing the eye.

Eyedrops. Some surgeons keep the pupil dilated with a daily cycloplegic or mydriatic eyedrop for one or two months. Others prefer to dilate only when the pupil appears to be constricting. The purpose of dilatation is to move the pupil (iris) enough that adhesions between the iris and the vitreous face do not form with the pupil in a constricted position. These adhesions would thus inhibit dilatation at any future time and would keep the pupil constricted. In addition, glaucoma may develop from blockage of aqueous flow into the anterior chamber. The buildup of aqueous

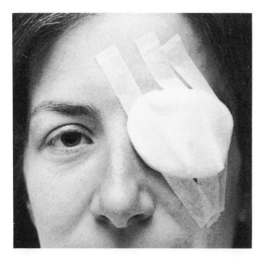

Figure 5–4. *Eyepatch. (Photo courtesy of Frank Flanagin, Associated Retinal Consultants, Detroit.)*

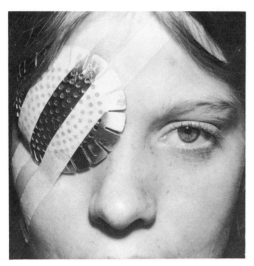

Figure 5–5. *Eyeshield. (Photo courtesy of Frank Flanagin, Associated Retinal Consultants, Detroit.)*

behind the iris will cause the iris to move forward and block the anterior chamber angle.

The type of intraocular lens that was implanted dictates the type of eyedrop to be instilled postoperatively. If an anterior chamber lens is implanted, then a mydriatic eyedrop is instilled. This dilatation prevents the complications of iritis and synechiae (adhesions) from occurring. If an iris plane lens is inserted, then a miotic type eyedrop is instilled. This constricts the pupil and prevents dislocation of the lens. With iris fixed (iris plane) lenses, dilating the pupil runs the risk of dislocating the lens either into the anterior chamber (which may cause corneal damage) or into the vitreous (which makes replacement very difficult). Three to five days postoperatively, if the surgeon feels synechiae are forming, he will cautiously dilate the eye with mydriatic.

Many surgeons use an antibiotic drop to prevent infection and some use a steroid eyedrop to reduce the postoperative inflammatory reaction.

Pain, Nausea, Vomiting. For one to two days postoperatively patients may have a scratching or itching reaction. This is a manifestation of pain and is usually relieved by an analgesic (Darvon) or a mild narcotic preparation (Empirin #3 or Tylenol No. 3).

Patients may have nausea and vomiting, and if so an antiemetic drug is given. If nausea and vomiting occur it is of short duration, usually only the day of surgery.

EYEGLASSES AND CONTACT LENSES

When the eyepatch is removed, the patient can be given a pair of temporary cataract glasses. These glasses are usually plus 10 diopters in strength, which is the approximate refracting power of the human lens. Therefore, these temporary glasses approximate the original focusing power of the eye.

These glasses are temporary because the patient eventually receives permanent glasses for accurate correction of the amount of refractive power loss of that eye. Because of the optics involved, this powerful +10 (convex lens) exerts a magnifying effect not present when the same power lens was in the eye.

Because of the magnifying effect, patients usually are warned to be careful when walking on stairs, when pouring hot coffee, or when attempting to sit down. Patients are told not to sit until they feel the chair behind their legs. Patients have difficulty with depth and distance perception but do adjust to this in time.

Patients who have intraocular lens implants do not have the problems of decreased visual field, magnification or loss of depth perception, and distance perception. The intraocular lens approximates the patient's normal lens. Patients may have a residual refractive error, and therefore need glasses to correct this error. These glasses are the "normal" lens and not the heavy cataract type lens.

The corneoscleral wound does not become completely healed for several months. The scar formation which occurs during this healing process affects the corneal curvature, and the curvature of the cornea has an effect on the final focusing of the eye. Therefore, permanent glasses or contact lenses are not given until approximately three months postoperatively, at which time the incision is completely healed.

There are several reasons that some patients prefer to wear contact lenses. A contact lens rests on the cornea, and because of the optical properties involved, it does not cause the same magnification as cataract glasses. In addition, the field of vision is greater with a contact lens. Following a unilateral cataract extraction, a contact lens usually must be used to prevent the magnification problems if both eyes are to be used simultaneously.

INFANTS WITH CONGENITAL CATARACTS

We know that the young infant with a visual disability such as congenital cataracts is receiving distorted views of his environment. Since each disability is unique, retardation in visual growth must be assessed individually. There are some points in visual growth and development that are pertinent to planning nursing care for the infant.

The 5- to 6-week-old baby appears to look at his mother's face and the hairline, but probably sees only form. By eight to nine weeks the baby is noticing his mother's eyes and thus is said to have developed a mental representation of what a human face looks like.

The new baby is said to be able to differentiate between light and dark. Babies have visual pursuit movements when only days old, and thus follow a brightly colored object. Seven to eight weeks pass before the infant has binocular fixation. At 16 weeks the baby is seen to begin to accommodate and focus on both near and far objects. However, this accommodation ability is not complete until the infant is four months old.

Cataract surgery may be performed as early as three months of age. This is the time when normally a baby smiles at a human face. However, it is felt that the baby is not responding to its mother. Attachment to the mother does not occur until around 7 months of age. Signs of separation grief for the mother then follow 1 month later.

Therefore, primary nursing care or, if possible, rooming in for the mother permits the baby to have support in a new and strange circumstance. The baby is petted, cooed to, rocked, and comforted. This will assist the baby to develop and deal with his surgery in a positive way, and, according to the advocates of attachment behavior, would be supportive care during this phase of the baby's life.

Postoperatively the baby's vital signs should be monitored. Protective mitts should be worn on the baby's arms and hands to prevent the infant from touching his eye dressings. Any increase in intraocular pressure should be prevented. Therefore, crying should be kept to a minimum. The rocking and patting of the baby by its mother during this time aids in preventing an increase in intraocular pressure.

Babies show sensitivity to pain by being irritable, crying, or by not sleeping well. If the baby is very irritable postoperatively and cries, frequently needing to be held and rocked, we may assume that he is uncomfortable. Some medication to relieve pain should be given. Also a barbiturate may be given to keep the baby relaxed and resting quietly.

Eyedrops or eye ointments will be ordered postoperatively. Usually steroid or antibiotic along with a dilating medication is instilled. Clean eyepatches and protective shields should be placed on the baby after each instillation of medication. Patching prevents irritation from light and thus may prevent some crying.

SELECTED READINGS

BOOKS

Bellows, J. G. *Cataract and Abnormalities of the Lens.* New York: Grune & Stratton, 1975.

Emery, J. M., and Patton, D. (Eds.). *Current Concepts in Cataract Surgery.* St. Louis: Mosby, 1974.

Jaffe, N. S. *Cataract Surgery and Its Complications* (2d ed.). St. Louis: Mosby, 1976.

Johnson, R. C., and Medinnus, G. R. *Child Psychology Behavior and Development* (3d ed.). New York: Wiley, 1974. Pp. 263–270.

McLean, J. *Atlas of Cataract Surgery*. St. Louis: Mosby, 1974.

Mussen, P. H., Conger, J. J., and Kagan, J. *Child Development and Personality* (4th ed.). New York: Harper & Row, 1974. P. 144.

ARTICLES

Boyd-Monk, H. Cataract surgery. *Nursing 77,* pp. 56–61, June 1977.

Smith, J. F. Focusing your care for the patient with an intraocular lens implant. *R.N.* 41(3): 46–87, 1978.

CHAPTER 6

THE VITREOUS BODY

ANATOMY

The vitreous body is a clear gel-like substance that fills the posterior portion of the eyeball. Its structure can be visualized as a meshwork frame of fine collagen fibers with the spaces filled by hyaluronic acid. Collagen is a protein and hyaluronic acid is a mucopolysaccharide. The fibrous network becomes more dense toward the outermost portion of the vitreous and is most dense in the areas of strong attachment between the vitreous and retina. These attachments occur at the optic disc and at the extreme anterior edge of the retina, the ora serrata (Fig. 6–1). Less firm vitreoretinal attachments occur at the macula and at the equator.

The fibrous network is most dense, and thus the gel consistency most thick, in the outer portion of the vitreous anteriorly. Although the vitreous is in approximation with the retina in all areas (in the eyes of the young), the 4- to 6-mm strip that straddles the ora serrata has the tightest adherence to the retina. This area is called the vitreous base. As the eye ages, the vitreous body collapses, and the areas formerly filled by vitreous are replaced by watery fluid much like aqueous. This collapse occurs in most of the population by the age of 60 years, but it can occur earlier in the presence of intraocular inflammation, myopia, or hemorrhage, or following surgery or trauma.

DISORDERS

DETACHMENT

When collapse does occur, the posterior vitreous peels away from its attachment to the retina and moves forward. This condition is called a *posterior vitreous detachment* (Fig. 6–2). The vitreous never, under natural circumstances, detaches from the vitreous base. Thus fastened anteriorly, the shrunken vitreous body floats in the watery fluid filling the remainder of the vitreous cavity.

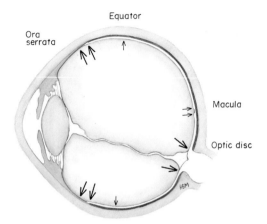

Figure 6–1. *Vitreous attachments.*

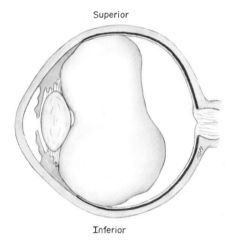

Figure 6–2. *Posterior vitreous detachment.*

This phenomenon gives rise to two symptoms that may exist together or independently.

Floaters

The most common symptom is that of "floaters." Floaters are the result of any thickening within the vitreous cavity. They occur because the thicker material blocks incoming light rays and casts a shadow on the retina. Any density will cause a floater, but the most common causes are coagulated vitreous and hemorrhage. Hemorrhage may occur when the adhesions between the posterior vitreous and the retina separate. Traction on the retinal blood vessels may cause momentary bleeding without apparent damage to the retina. These bleeding sites are rarely able to be seen unless a retinal tear occurs at the time. Floaters are noticed by the patient only when the densities lie close to the central visual axis (the direct line extending outward from the macula through the center of the pupil). The farther an opacity lies from this line, the less likely that it will cause symptoms. It is common for a patient to describe floaters when his eyes are in a certain position but not at other times. Most of these floaters, whatever their cause, will diminish or disappear over weeks to months, but some remain indefinitely. Other than time, no effective treatment for floaters exists.

Light Flashes

The other symptom of posterior vitreous detachment is that of light flashes. Light flashes occur as a result of tugging by the moving vitreous body on its retinal attachments. Since the retina can react to stimulation in only one manner, that of light sensation, light flashes occur most frequently when the vitreous body is in stages of active change. These flashes are usually very subtle and are most often described as lightning flashes occurring when the patient is in a dark room. They tend to last for a relatively short period of time—days to weeks—in most people. Probably these flashes occur at some time in everyone but, since they are of such short duration, they are rationalized as being from an extraneous light source and are rapidly forgotten.

Floaters and flashes are commonly associated with retinal detachments. (See Chap. 7, Retinal Holes, p. 200.) Retinal detachment or retinal tear must be considered in the presence of such symptoms, and a thorough evaluation of the peripheral retina should be performed.

HEMORRHAGE

Massive vitreous hemorrhage may occur secondary to any retinal disease associated with abnormal retinal blood vessels. The most common diseases affecting the retina in this fashion are diabetes, sickle cell anemia, retinal vein occlusion, and various congenital retinal vascular abnormalities. Massive hemorrhage can also occur at the time of a posterior vitreous detachment or of the development of a retinal hole. Most of these hemorrhages will be absorbed in time. Some will coagulate and cause traction between the vitreous and the retina, often leading to retinal detachment.

INFECTIONS OF THE MEMBRANES

Vitreous membranes may develop following any disturbance of the vitreous body whether before or after its normal collapse. These membranes are particularly common following inflammation in the choroid or retina and following intraocular penetration of a foreign material or laceration of the wall of the eye. Contraction of these membranes often results in traction on the retina, leading to vitreous hemorrhage or retinal detachment.

INFECTIONS

Infections of the vitreous are rare. More commonly, an infection of the retina or choroid will spread into the vitreous. When this happens, heroic measures are necessary to save the eye. Topical antibiotics will not penetrate into the vitreous cavity. Therefore, large doses of intravenous antibiotics and subconjunctival injections of the appropriate antibiotic are necessary. Recently, there has been greater interest in using intravitreal injections of antibiotics for severe cases of vitreitis and endophthalmitis. Several reports in the literature attest to the effectiveness of this treatment.

FOREIGN BODIES

Intravitreal foreign bodies have become less common as awareness of this problem has increased within industry. Most major manufacturing plants have safety programs that include safety glass requirements. Fifty years ago, many hospitals in areas with a large concentration of heavy industry might see several cases of intraocular foreign bodies every day. Now it is unusual to see one a week. The industrial nurse who sees a patient with a suspected intraocular foreign body should patch the eye and immediately send the patient to an ophthalmologist. The patient generally can tell the nurse that something has hit his eye. This should alert the industrial nurse to the possibility of an intraocular foreign body, particularly if the patient has been hammering or has been

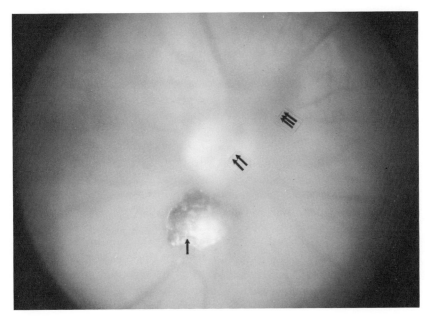

Figure 6–3. *Intravitreal foreign body. Single arrow points to foreign body. (Note glistening appearance of steel foreign body because of reflection of camera light flash.) Double arrow points to disc; triple arrow points to vitreal hemorrhage. (Photo courtesy of Frank Flanagin, Associated Retinal Consultants, Detroit.)*

adjacent to heavy machinery and thus subject to being hit by flying particles.

The foreign body is usually not found in the anterior chamber. It is most commonly in the vitreous cavity and thus can be seen only by using an ophthalmoscope (Fig. 6–3). However, careful evaluation of the anterior part of the eye may show one of the following: (1) a localized area of conjunctival injection and edema, often with a central conjunctival defect or laceration, (2) a corneal laceration, (3) a flat anterior chamber (this is almost always associated with a large corneal laceration), (4) a hole in the iris, (5) a hyphema, (6) evidence of cataract or other disturbance of the lens.

All of the above indicate tissue disturbance caused by a foreign body passing through various tissues. It is not uncommon for the eye to be quite comfortable and for the vision to be normal following intraocular penetration of a foreign body. Thus, the nurse must alert herself on the basis of history.

Intravitreal or intraocular foreign bodies usually should be removed. Glass and lead and a few other materials often are tolerated
by the eye. But the most common foreign bodies, iron and copper,
are poorly tolerated, and breakdown products of the metal almost
invariably lead to degeneration of the retina, if not destruction
of the entire eye. The foreign body is localized by x-ray. Several
methods can be used to outline the surface of the eye by radi-
opaque markers (e.g., the marked contact lens). The position of the
foreign body is determined by measuring from the markers, and
plotting the measurements on a special graph.

Iron and steel foreign bodies are removed by using a magnet.
An incision is made through the sclera usually over the foreign
body as localized by x-ray and ophthalmoscopy. This localization
can often be confirmed at surgery by using the magnet to pull
the foreign body toward the sclera and distorting the sclera at the
foreign body site. The scleral incision is made at that point. The
scleral incision is then spread and the foreign body pulled through
the retina and choroid using the magnet. A small amount of
vitreous usually escapes at the moment of removal. Because a
hole is made in the retina at the removal site, diathermy or cryothermy applications are placed to surround the removal site and
form a scar around the hole. Removal of a nonmagnetic foreign
body is much more hazardous and requires manipulation within
the vitreous cavity with a forceps to grasp the foreign body and
remove it. The techniques vary considerably, depending on the
position and size of the foreign body and the condition of the eye.

SURGERY

Over the last decade, new techniques have been developed to en-
able the surgeon to work in the vitreous cavity and remove diseased
vitreous. The original procedures were designed to cut the abnormal vitreous bands that caused retinal detachments. Now, however, most of the vitreous body can be removed and replaced with
a balanced salt solution.

The procedure that has become the most useful and the most
reliable is called the *pars plana vitrectomy.* Its performance depends on a special type of instrument (Fig. 6–4). There are many
designs available, but they all work essentially the same way (i.e.,
they suck vitreous or vitreous membranes, or vitreous hemorrhage
into a porthole in a needle about the size of an 18-gauge needle

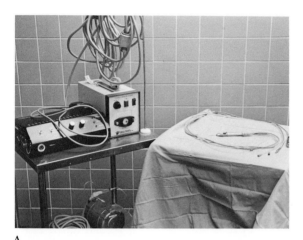

A

B

Figure 6–4. *Vitrectomy unit. A. The vitrectomy hand piece and its connections lie on the table. An electric motor within the cylindrical handle drives the cutter and is controlled through the black power box by a foot pedal (on top of box). Intraocular illumination is provided by a fiber-optic sleeve over the needle. The light source is in the white-faced box. The remaining silicone tubes are for fluid inflow and outflow. B. Close-up of handpiece. (Photo courtesy of Frank Flanagin, Associated Retinal Consultants, Detroit.)*

and cut the material by means of a rotating or chopping movement by a sleeve inside the needle). The needle actually is double walled, and its other chamber has a second porthole, to allow inflow of a balanced salt solution that will replace the removed vitreous (Fig. 6–5). Suction is applied with the use of a syringe or by suction built into the machine. Inflow is usually regulated by gravity flow from a bottle hung as an intravenous bottle on a

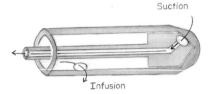

Figure 6–5. *Vitrectomy unit. Tip of vitrectomy instrument showing saline inflow (infusion) port and suction or cutting port. Cutting is accomplished by rotation of the inner piece.*

stand. Intraocular pressure can be varied by changing the height of the bottle. The procedure is performed by inserting the cutting needle of the instrument through a 3 mm incision in the pars plana into the vitreous cavity. Visualization is achieved with the operating microscope and a corneal contact lens. After all the diseased vitreous is removed, the instrument is withdrawn from the eye and the incision closed with several interrupted sutures. The result can be elimination of all diseased vitreous or hemorrhage and its replacement with a clear balanced salt solution. This solution will eventually be replaced by an aqueous fluid produced by the eye.

The vitrectomy operation is most useful in the management of diabetic retinopathy with vitreous hemorrhage and traction detachments. It is also helpful in cases of retinal detachment with vitreous contraction, particularly those associated with vitreous hemorrhage and those secondary to trauma.

PREOPERATIVE NURSING CARE

The diabetic patient who is admitted for a vitrectomy is generally seen by an endocrinologist or internist before surgery. There then is the opportunity to determine fasting blood glucose levels if the patient is a diabetic and to do the routine laboratory work. This generally consists of a complete blood count, determination of hematocrit and hemoglobin levels, and a chest x-ray. If the patient is over 40 years of age, an ECG is taken.

Apprehension and anxiety should be allayed by giving explanations for hospital procedures. The patients may or may not have been hospitalized previously. Some of these patients may have had previous retinal detachment surgery. Others may have been treated for other retinal conditions. Hence patient familiarity with hospitals varies.

Usually the patient's vision is poor. A large number of patients having vitrectomy surgery will have vision of less than 20/200; hence, by definition, the patient is legally blind. Because of the decreased vision, safety precautions are essential. Care of the blind should be instituted when it is applicable to the patient's safety and visual status.

The patient needs orientation to his immediate environment. Personal belongings such as robe and slippers should be left in a place where they can be readily found. Nurses frequently move slippers and robes when caring for the patient, hence making it difficult for them to be relocated without calling hospital personnel for assistance. Since the patient is adjusted to having poor vision he generally is able to move about the room. Hospital policies vary, and some institutions prefer to have the patient call for a nurse before going to the bathroom, or venturing out of bed independently.

The pupil is dilated with a mydriatic and cycloplegic eyedrop. The mydriatic can be a drug such as phenylephrine hydrochloride (Neo-Synephrine 10%); the cycloplegic can be a drug such as cyclopentolate hydrochloride (Cyclogyl 1%), atropine 1%, scopolamine 0.25%, or homatropine. This dilatation achieves two purposes: it permits the availability of examining the retina at any time; and it prevents the iritis that is frequently associated with intraocular surgery from binding the pupil in a constricted state and thus prohibiting any future dilatation of that pupil.

Preoperative medications vary with the individual surgeon. Usually a narcotic, a sedative, and a narcotic potentiator or tranquilizer are given. An example of a frequently given preoperative medication would be meperidine (Demerol) 75 mg and hydroxyzine pamoate (Vistaril) 50 mg given intramuscularly one hour preoperatively. Pentobarbital (Nembutal) 100 mg orally is given 1½ hours preoperatively. Atropine is given intramuscularly to reduce secretions if the patient is to have a general anesthetic.

A mydriatic and cycloplegic eyedrop are instilled preoperatively as well as an antibiotic eyedrop to reduce the pathogens in the conjunctiva.

POSTOPERATIVE NURSING CARE

Postoperative nursing care is the same as for any surgical patient. Vital signs of blood pressure, pulse, and respirations should be taken every 15 minutes until the patient is stable then once every shift for 24 hours.

Patients return from surgery with one or both eyes patched. The operated eye is always patched for cleanliness and patient comfort. Some surgeons prefer to patch both eyes following surgery. The theory is that if both eyes are patched they will be at rest and there will be less postoperative inflammation.

Safety precautions are essential if binocular patching is used. Assistance with all aspects of nursing care is indicated. An explanation of the immediate environment is indicated if the patient has not had this previously, but since vision was probably poor preoperatively, he will have already had this orientation.

Saline or air is injected into the vitreous cavity to act as a mechanical agent to restore normal intraocular pressure. If saline is used, the patient does not have to be positioned in any particular manner. If some hemorrhage or bleeding persists the patient is placed in a semi-Fowler's position. This position (with the head of the bed slightly elevated) aids in permitting the blood to settle inferiorly and thus be below the visual axis.

Gas (e.g., air) may be used when some retinal detachment is present at the end of the operation. The patient is positioned so that the gas will mechanically press the retina into position. Since gas rises, the patient is positioned so that the area of the retina that needs to be flattened is uppermost. The surgeon, therefore, should designate head position because the affected area varies. If the area to be affected by the gas is at the posterior pole of the eye the patient may be flat (prone position) with a pillow or folded blanket under his chest and head; the face may be turned down slightly from the face-down position. Since this position must be maintained for four or five days, until the gas is absorbed, it becomes tedious and tiring for the patient. The nurse needs to remember that the patient can be in any position as long as the head remains face down and the gas is at the posterior pole. Therefore, the patient can sit in a Fowler's position, with his head resting on an overbed table, which can be adjusted for the patient's height. In changing position, the patient regains the desired position by placing his head face downward, which then causes the gas to rise to the back of the eye, and he then turns his head slightly, for comfort. Aphakic patients who have gas injected into the vitreous cavity should never lie on their backs for long periods of time. This position would cause the gas to rise, pushing the iris forward and closing the angle, thus causing an acute glaucoma. Patients who are not aphakic should avoid lying on their backs for long periods of time because gas in contact with the lens may cause a cataract.

Patients are permitted to be out of the desired position for short periods of time, such as to go to the bathroom or to sit and eat their meals. The desired position is always regained as described previously by lying in the prone position, (face downward) and then rotating the head slightly to a position of comfort.

Deep breathing is begun 15 times every hour if the patient has had a general anesthetic or if gas has been instilled. Patients who have had gas instilled have a tendency to lie quietly and tensely without moving. Taking deep breaths assists in relaxing the patient. Passive and active range of motion exercises are utilized to prevent the formation of thrombi. These exercises are also helpful for the patient with gas instillation. It aids in relaxing the tense patient and preventing him from lying in a motionless state and contracting his muscles, thereby becoming more susceptible to any manifestations of an anxious state. Because patients are generally anxious over their visual problems, these exercises aid in physical relaxation. The activity also gives the nurse an opportunity to talk with the patient and hence to assist in answering questions or help him to avoid the boredom and loneliness that hospitalization can bring.

If patients are bilaterally patched, we generally try to visit the patient five minutes out of every hour. We encourage the patient to listen to the news, a favorite talk show, or musical program to assist him in remaining oriented, and to keep from being bored and day dreaming. We ask patients to use their memory to assist in orientation by telling us what they heard on the newscasts.

Postoperative dilatation of the pupil is maintained with a mydriatic and cycloplegic. Another eyedrop, an antibiotic and corticosteroid, is given to reduce inflammation and to lower pathogens in the conjunctiva. These drops are instilled four times a day.

Edema and discomfort of the eyelids vary with individuals. When removing the eyepatch to instill the eyedrops, you may see the eyes and eyelids so swollen that the conjunctiva is edematous and is peeking through the swollen lids. This may frighten the inexperienced nurse who feels that something has surely gone amiss. There may be a moderate amount of drainage for 24 to 48 hours postoperatively. Cold compresses are ordered at least four times a day to relieve this chemosis and ecchymosis as well as for lid comfort and cleanliness. Patching the eye and keeping it at rest also assists in reducing this edema.

Pain or discomfort in the operative eye varies. Frequently patients describe this pain as a temporal or frontal headache. Medications vary depending on severity of discomfort. Meperidine (Demerol) 50 to 100 mg, acetaminophen with codeine (Tylenol) 325 mg. per tablet, one or two tablets, or Tylenol gr 10 are administered as needed to give relief.

Postoperative nausea and vomiting vary with individual patients. An antiemetic is ordered and generally suffices to relieve the discomfort.

Discharge teaching should begin on the first postoperative day or at the earliest possible time. Discharge usually is seven to ten days after surgery. Physicians generally request patients to come for a postoperative visit one week after discharge. Patients are discharged with two eyedrops—a cycloplegic and an anti-inflammatory, antibiotic type drop to be instilled four times a day.

During the second week after surgery, any activity that would cause an increase in venous hypertension (e.g., heavy exercise, Valsalva maneuver) should be avoided. The patient may be up and about at home, watching television and reading.

Patient vision can be excellent if the retina has not been damaged. If the patient has suffered retinal damage, vision can be very poor.

SELECTED READINGS

BOOKS

Krill, A. E. *Krill's Hereditary Retinal and Choroidal Diseases. Vol. 2, Clinical Characteristics.* Hagerstown, MD: Harper & Row, 1977.
Pruett, R. C., Regan, C. D. J. *Retinal Congress.* New York: Appleton-Century-Crofts, 1972.

ARTICLE

Stone, R. D. Vitrectomy. *Western Journal of Medicine,* 126(2): 127–128, 1977.

CHAPTER 7 ⸻

RETINA, CHOROID, AND
OPTIC NERVE

The retina, choroid, and optic nerve will be considered together because the diseases that affect one usually involve one or both of the others (Fig. 7–1).

ANATOMY

RETINA

The retina is the innermost layer of the wall of the eye. It is approximately 0.2 to 0.4 mm in thickness and covers the entire posterior portion of the eye, extending forward to a level about 7 mm behind the corneal limbus. The retina is divided into two layers called the *retinal pigment epithelium* and the *retinal neuroepithelium*. The pigment epithelium is a single layer of epithelial cells on the external side of the retina. The neuroepithelium is a multilayered structure of nerve elements; it is also called the *sensory retina*. A retinal detachment is a collapse of the neuroepithelium only, and the splitting occurs at the level of neuroepithelium and pigment epithelium.

Histologically, the retina is divided into several levels (Fig. 7–2). The visual cells, the rods and cones, comprise the outermost layer and rest against the retinal pigment epithelium. The second level, neurons, are bipolar cells that form connections between the visual cells and the innermost layer of cells, the ganglion cells; the bipolar cells also form connections between individual cells in the rod-and-cone layer. The axons of the ganglion cells form the nerve fiber layer of the retina and then join and form the optic nerve.

Clinically the major landmarks of the retina are the macula and optic disc (Fig. 7–3). The macula is a roughly oval area, about 1.5 mm in horizontal dimension, positioned at the center of the posterior part of the eye. The innermost retinal elements are tilted away from the center in the macular area, thinning the retina slightly and giving better exposure to the visual cell layer in this

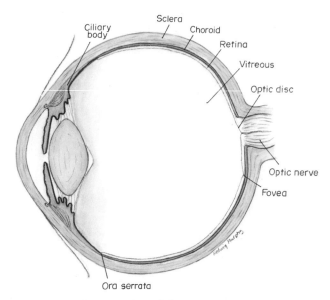

Figure 7–1. *Cross section of the eye.*

thinner area. The visual cells here are almost entirely cones—the site of the sharp discriminating vision, which is cone vision.

The optic disc is approximately 2 to 3 mm (1.5 to 2 disc diameters) nasal to the macula and is about 1.5 mm in diameter. The optic disc is the anterior surface of the optic nerve. Axons of all the ganglion cells in the retina extend toward the optic disc and form the optic nerve at the optic disc. The retinal blood vessels begin branching into the retina at the optic disc.

The visual cells in the periphery are almost entirely rods. Therefore, since the function of the rods is mainly perception of light and dark, and the function of the cones is mostly fine discrimination and color discrimination, the retinal periphery has better capability to recognize light intensity and also rapid movement. The macula, on the other hand, functions as the site of fine discrimination and color vision.

The process by which vision occurs is complicated, but there are several essential changes that must occur. For light to strike the visual organ and be absorbed, a pigment capable of absorbing light is required. Then, a chemical process must occur, which results in an electrical nervous impulse being formed. In the process, the products of the chemical reaction must be removed (other-

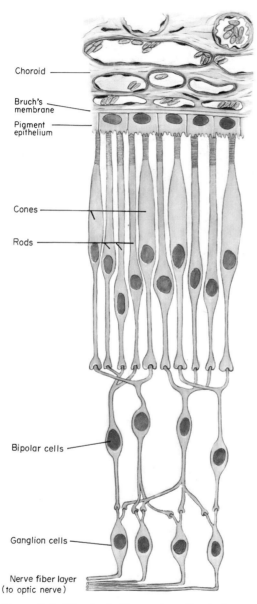

Figure 7-2. *Histologic illustration of retinal cells.*

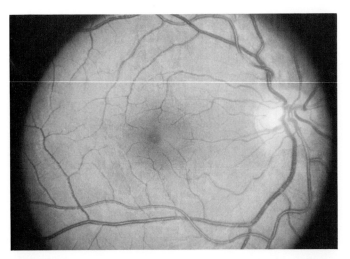

Figure 7-3. *Normal macula and disc. (Photo courtesy of Frank Flanagin, Associated Retinal Consultants, Detroit.)*

wise the image would persist), and the photochemical substance must be capable of regeneration.

This photochemical substance, a protein called *rhodopsin* or *visual purple,* has been isolated from the retina. This substance, when exposed to light, bleaches to a pale orangish color. From this pigment a vitamin A derivative, retinene, can be isolated. Further bleaching causes reduction of the vitamin A aldehyde to vitamin A. The entire process is reversible in the presence of the proper enzymes and chemicals. This chemical reaction would fit the requirements that we have postulated as necessary to produce a visual image.

CHOROID

The choroid consists mainly of blood vessels roughly divided into three layers. The outer layer is of large vessels, the middle layer is of medium-sized vessels, and the inner layer (choriocapillaris) consists of large-bore capillaries packed very close together so that the effect is that of a large lake of blood. The outer two layers also have a significant amount of pigment scattered between the vessels, but the choriocapillaris does not. There is an inner lamina which is a thin, structureless membrane forming the inner bound-

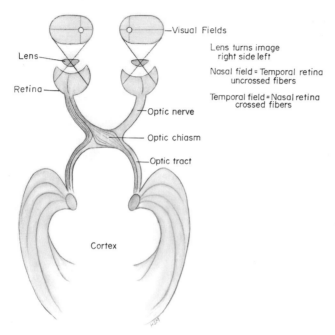

Lens—
Retina—

—Visual Fields

Lens turns image
right side left

Nasal field = Temporal retina
uncrossed fibers

Temporal field = Nasal retina
crossed fibers

—Optic nerve

— Optic chiasm

—Optic tract

Cortex

Figure 7–4. *The relationship between visual field, retina, and
optic nerve. Note that each area of visual field is served by
retina on the opposite side of the eye. Note that the left visual
cortex serves the right visual field of each eye, and vice versa.*

ary of choroid, which is called Bruch's membrane. It is adjacent
to the outer side of the retinal pigment epithelium.

The function of the choroid is to supply nutrition to the retinal
rod-and-cone-layer, which does not receive significant blood supply from the retinal vessels.

OPTIC NERVE

The optic nerve is formed from the axons of the ganglion cells of
the retina. Each optic nerve passes out of its respective orbit,
where it joins with the optic nerve from the other side in a crossing
structure called the *optic chiasm* (Fig. 7–4). At the optic chiasm,
the fibers from the inner side of each retina cross and the fibers
from the outer side of each retina remain on their respective
sides. The continuation of the crossed nerve fibers behind the
optic chiasm is called the *optic tract,* which carries impulses to
the brain.

Injuries to the nerve supply can be localized on the basis of whether they cause damage to the visual field in each eye or whether they cause damage to the visual field of only one eye. Since an area of the retina affects the visual field on the opposite side (that is, the right half of the retina in the right eye produces the left half of the visual field of the right eye), damage to the right optic tract will cause a loss of visual field on the left side of each eye, whereas damage to the right optic nerve will cause loss of visual field on both sides of the right eye.

SPECIAL DIAGNOSTIC INSTRUMENTS AND TESTS

OPHTHALMOSCOPE

The universally used instrument for study of the retina is, of course, the ophthalmoscope. Actually there are two types of ophthalmoscopes—direct and indirect. The direct ophthalmoscope, which is the common type of ophthalmoscope used by all physicians, gives an upright image of the retina and covers an area approximately 2 disc diameters in diameter (Fig. 7–5). It has the advantage of high magnification, about 15 power. The indirect ophthalmoscope gives a totally inverted image. It is difficult to get as much magnification with the indirect ophthalmoscope, but a greater field of vision is possible, so that one may see areas up to 10 or more disc diameters in diameter at one time. The advantage of this instrument is that it allows one to "see the forest rather than the trees." If an abnormality is noted which needs to be examined under higher magnification, the direct ophthalmoscope can be used.

SCLERAL DEPRESSOR

A scleral depressor is used in conjunction with the indirect ophthalmoscope by most examiners. As the name implies, the purpose is to indent the scleral surface at the anterior portion of the retina. This pushes the retina toward the pupil and allows areas normally hidden behind the iris to be seen. The depressor itself is a small, blunt-tipped metal or plastic rod (Fig. 7–6). Pressure can be exerted on the lid or directly on the sclera. If the scleral depressor is used properly, the patient experiences very little, if any, discomfort.

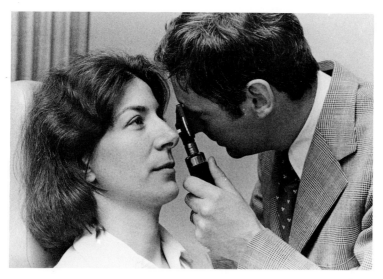

Figure 7–5. *Patient being examined with direct ophthalmoscope. (Photo courtesy of Frank Flanagin, Associated Retinal Consultants, Detroit.)*

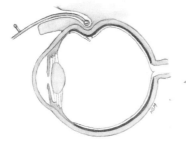

Figure 7–6. *Scleral depression through the lid. In this illustration the indentation is localized on a retinal tear.*

CONTACT LENS

Another method of examining the retina employs a contact lens on the surface of the cornea to convert the curved surface of the cornea to the flat surface of the contact lens. The examination is performed with a slit lamp looking through the contact lens (Fig. 7–7). The examiner can then look through the pupil as if he were looking through a window.

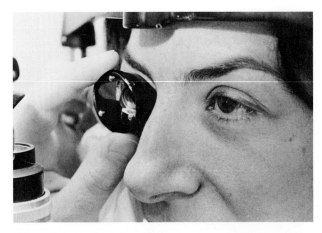

Figure 7–7. *Retinal examination using contact lens and a slit lamp. (Photo courtesy of Frank Flanagin, Associated Retinal Consultants, Detroit.)*

PHOTOGRAPHY

Retinal photography has become popular over the last two to three decades (Fig. 7–8). With the advent of improved light sources and film, photography is now a rapid and useful method of documenting retinal changes. In addition, angiography of the retinal blood vessels can be performed by using appropriate filters, black-and-white film, and fluorescein dye injected into the antecubital vein. The result is a black-and-white photograph that has all the appearances of an x-ray arteriogram. Rapid sequence photography will document the retinal blood flow. Photographs are usually taken at approximately one-second intervals. A timer registers the time on the photograph so that arm-to-eye circulation and retinal arteriovenous circulation times can be evaluated. The injection is made rapidly and the timer started simultaneously. The dye normally appears in the retinal arteries 10 to 16 sec after injection. The veins are usually completely filled within 25 sec. Rapid-sequence photos at 1/sec are taken from about 9 sec after injection until about 30 secs. Photos are taken again, usually at one and five minutes (Fig. 7–9). Occasionally it is helpful to obtain photos about one hour later.

The pupil must be dilated to perform the retinal photography procedure. Fluorescein angiography is a safe procedure but occasionally allergic reactions occur. These are usually limited to itch-

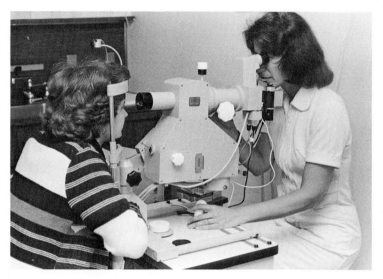

Figure 7-8. *Fundus camera. Photographer is on the right. (Photo courtesy of Frank Flanagin, Associated Retinal Consultants, Detroit.)*

ing and hives. Intense burning occurs if the dye leaks subcutaneously. Usually short-acting cycloplegics (Cyclogyl or Mydriacyl) are used in combination with Neo-Synephrine (a powerful but short-acting mydriatic) to obtain maximum pupil dilatation.

ULTRASONOGRAPHY

Ultrasonography has become extremely helpful in determining gross outline changes in the retina and choroid in eyes that have cloudy corneas or lenses, which prevent fundus examination. This test has become very sophisticated within the last five years, so that excellent demonstration of major pathology within the eye can be performed (Fig. 7-10). Such lesions as retinal detachment, choroidal and retinal tumors, and fibrous tissue proliferations can easily be documented.

ELECTRORETINOGRAPHY

Electroretinography is the process of graphing the measurement of the retina's electric response to light stimulation. Lights at varying speeds and varying intensities are flashed, and the nervous response is graphed in a manner similar to that of electrocardiography or electroencephalography (Fig. 7-11). Electroretinography

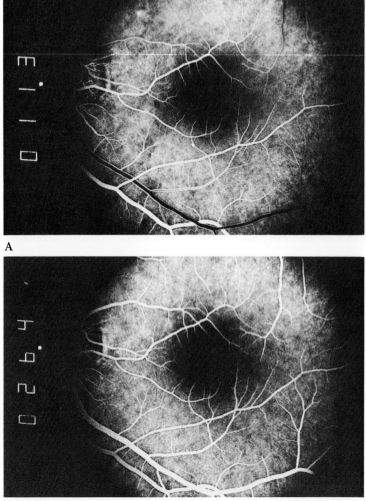

B
Figure 7-9. *Fluorescein angiography. The numbers at left indicate time after injection. A. Arteries are filled and veins just beginning to fill. B. Veins completely filled.*

is particularly helpful in evaluating widespread degenerative retinal diseases. It is less helpful in evaluating localized lesions, even lesions causing marked decreased vision, such as a large scar involving the entire macula. It can be helpful in evaluating the visual

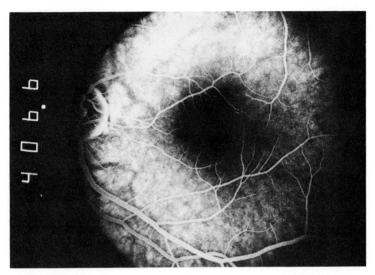

C

Figure 7-9. (continued) *C. Late picture showing the choroid well filled with fluorescein.*

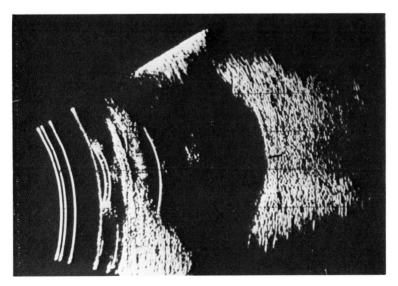

Figure 7-10. *B-scan ultrasonogram. Arrow points to the posterior inner wall of the globe. Its smooth surface indicates no mass or gross disturbance of the retina.*

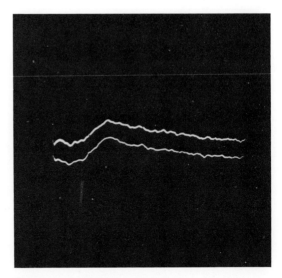

Figure 7–11. *Electroretinogram.*

potential of an eye with a severe cataract if the vision is markedly reduced.

RADIOACTIVE ISOTOPES

Phosphorus 32 radioactive isotope studies have gained renewed interest in application to intraocular tumors. These studies have been particularly helpful in the differential diagnosis of elevated choroidal lesions. The difference between choroidal hemorrhage and choroidal tumor can almost invariably be interpreted by this test. The test involves giving the patient a measured amount of the isotope phosphorus 32. After 48 hours, a small Geiger counter is placed on the surface of the sclera and counts are taken over the lesion and then over a normal area. An elevation of the number of counts in the area of the lesion indicates that a malignant tumor is present. This test has been more than 95 percent accurate when performed properly. If the suspected lesion is anterior to the equator, the count may be performed through the conjunctiva. If the lesion is posterior to the equator, a conjunctival incision must be made. In either case, accurate localization of the tumor is essential, because application of the counter as little as 2 mm from the lesion may result in a negative result.

INFECTIONS AND INFLAMMATIONS

The choroid and retina are closely adherent, and any significant infection or inflammation involving the choroid invariably effects the retina to a greater or lesser degree. In addition, the choroid is only one division of the uvea, which is comprised of the iris, ciliary body, and choroid. These divisions are developmentally similar and structurally contiguous so that they all respond to inflammation in one division, although not with equal intensity.

In spite of this, certain diseases do have a predilection for certain divisions of the uvea and we will direct our remarks to some of those effects on the choroid and retina.

UVEITIS

The pathology is relatively similar in all types of choroiditis. In the early stages, there is infiltration by polymorphonuclear leukocytes, lymphocytes, and fibrin in the affected area. As progression occurs, the inflammatory material breaks into the retina and then, in the more active diseases, lesions involve the vitreous. In chronic uveitis, mononuclear cells predominate. Usually these lesions are rather well circumscribed, and, more often than not, they do not involve the macula. The final result is a white scar, demonstrating destruction of the choroid and overlying retina in that area.

Symptoms are related to the site of the inflammation and to the effects of the inflammatory products that make their way into the vitreous. The vitreous debris will cause blurred vision and floaters, which may be the only symptom. These floaters usually absorb with time, and the only visual defect is caused by the choroidal (chorioretinal) scar. If this scar is in the macula, the magnitude of the visual defect can be very great. However, if it is not, as is more often the case, vision may return to normal. Light flashes may occur secondary to vitreous contraction and vitreoretinal traction. The conjunctiva is often injected. There may be light sensitivity because of the iritis.

The most common causes of posterior uveitis now recognized are toxoplasmosis and histoplasmosis.

Toxoplasmosis

Toxoplasma gondii is an intracellular parasite that invades and multiplies within the host cell until the cell bursts. If the cell

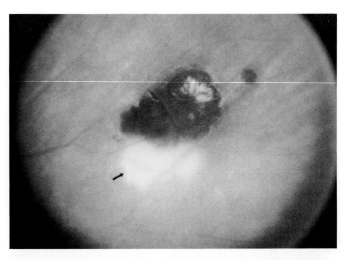

Figure 7-12. *Toxoplasmosis scarring. Black area indicates dormant chorioretinal scar. Arrow points to reactivated lesion adjacent to old scar. (Photo courtesy of Frank Flanagin, Associated Retinal Consultants, Detroit.)*

resists the multiplying process, the parasite forms a pseudocyst with multiple parasites. The pseudocysts may reactivate later. All organs of the body may be invaded, but the eye is a common site and the chorioretinal scar from toxoplasmosis is very dense (Fig. 7-12).

The disease may be encountered during fetal life if the mother becomes infected during pregnancy. If the involvement occurs during the early stages of pregnancy, abortion will usually result. In later stages, severe infections may lead to splenomegaly, hydrocephalus, cerebral calcification, mental retardation, and so on. Milder infections may demonstrate few systemic signs, but ocular lesions are present in over 10 percent of the congenitally infected. It is rare for the fetus to acquire the disease if the mother has been infected prior to the pregnancy, even if reactivation occurs during pregnancy. Thus, an old chorioretinal scar in the mother is almost a guarantee against the fetus being infected.

Whether congenital or acquired, the parasite settles in the retina and causes severe necrosis, which invariably leads to chorioretinal infiltration, edema, and vitreous exudate. Usually, the process is self limited but encysted parasites may cause reactivation of the lesion at a later date. The vast majority of active *Toxoplasmosis* seen in adults is the result of reactivation of congenital lesions. The final scar is white with pigment usually at the periphery of the scar. If reactivation occurs, it occurs at the edge of the previous scar.

T. gondii is transmitted to humans who come in contact with oocytes in infected cat feces. Usually a presumptive diagnosis can be made clinically. A positive titer of any level by one of the serum dye tests is considered confirmatory.

Treatment is initiated only if the lesion threatens the macula or if the inflammatory process runs unabated for several months. Usually, the process subsides spontaneously within six weeks, although it may take longer for the vitreous debris to be absorbed. Pyrimethamine (Daraprim) combined with sulfonamides is the treatment of choice. However, pyrimethamine frequently causes bone marrow toxicity. The initial sign of toxicity is depression in the circulating platelets, and therefore weekly platelet counts should be performed. The toxicity can be prevented by the concomitant use of folinic acid. Lincomycin has recently been demonstrated to be effective and may supplant Daraprim.

Histoplasmosis

Histoplasmosis is a fungus disease and is particularly prevalent in the Mississippi Valley in the United States. The systemic infection is usually very mild, often like a mild upper respiratory infection. It is rare to see the initial acute chorioretinal involvement. The choroiditis leaves several to many small (less than one disc diameter), white, punched out disk-like lesions, most of which are in the midperiphery. These lesions may develop within the macular area, but they do not affect the vision even if they are adjacent to the macula. However, the lesions near the macula will often reactivate and develop subretinal neovascularization, subretinal hemorrhage, and scarring in the macula, causing serious loss of macular vision. Pigmented peripapillary atrophy is usually present. The diagnostic triad includes punched out peripheral scars, submacular hemorrhage or scar, and peripapillary atrophy (Fig. 7–13).

Treatment is not necessary unless the hemorrhagic phase occurs. Then photocoagulation of the active lesion is frequently successful. This can be performed only if the lesion is discovered before it progresses closer than 0.25 disc diameter to the macula. Otherwise the photocoagulation scar itself will damage the macula. Oral or

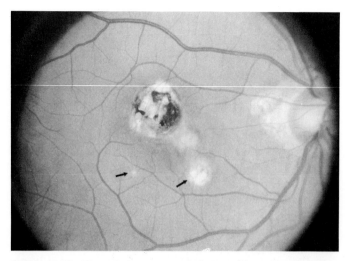

Figure 7–13. *Histoplasmosis. Typical triad of presumed ocular histoplasmosis chorioretinitis: Macular scar, perimacular and/or peripheral punched out lesions (arrows), and atrophy around disc. (Photo courtesy of Frank Flanagin, Associated Retinal Consultants, Detroit.)*

subconjunctival steroids have also been used to combat this hemorrhagic phase with variable success. They must often be used in high doses for a year or more.

Unfortunately, a high percentage of patients who develop macular lesions in one eye will later develop the same progression in the other eye. This likelihood is very great if the small disc lesions are discovered in the perimacular area. These patients should be observed closely and warned to return for immediate evaluation if any visual distortion should develop, since pain and acute signs of inflammation do not occur. Activation of the second eye may occur 10 to 20 years after that of the first eye. No preventive therapy is known.

CHORIORETINITIS

Tuberculous and syphilitic chorioretinitis have become rare as the systemic diseases have been controlled. Tuberculous chorioretinitis is usually seen in the miliary form of the systemic disease, particularly in young patients. The choroidal disease demonstrates many yellowish-white, dense spots, about one disc diameter in size, most often seen in the posterior pole. Less common is the finding of a large patchy lesion. These lesions consist of giant cells and mononuclear cells. Tubercle bacilli can be recovered from the lesions.

Treatment requires appropriate antituberculous therapy using isoniazid (INH) and para-aminosalicylic acid (PAS). Judicious use of corticosteroids may also be indicated.

Acquired syphilitic chorioretinitis is usually not seen until the secondary stage or the late tertiary stage of the systemic disease. It is usually associated with iritis and demonstrates either patchy or confluent yellowish chorioretinal lesions. There is often significant vitreous reaction. The late-stage disease has a less explosive onset but the lesions are quite similar. The pathology is similar, demonstrating intense inflammatory response, beginning in the choriocapillaris, which breaks into the retina and involves all layers of retina and choroid. The result is many discrete or large multifocal scars.

Congenital syphilis is more likely to cause a widespread salt-and-pepper-like degeneration. However, almost any chorioretinal degenerative process may be mimicked.

Serological studies of serum and spinal fluid should be performed. However, because syphilis can occur even in serologically negative patients, negative findings should not rule out the presence of disease.

Treatment should include specific antisyphilitic antibiotics. Systemic steroids are usually necessary.

Toxocara canis and *cati* are uncommon but not rare. The parasite eggs are eliminated in dog and cat feces and ingested by youngsters, particularly those who are dirt eaters. The parasite then travels to the eye and causes an intense inflammatory reaction, which at times is severe enough to obscure completely the posterior segment of the eye. If the eye is not destroyed, a prominent scar, often elevated, remains. If the scar is a reasonable distance from the macula, central vision may be spared; however, it is not uncommon for the scar at the inflammation site to cause retinal traction at another site and seriously affect vision. Often, the systemic disease is very mild, and diagnosis is difficult. Since the larva does not develop into the adult worm in man, search for worms or ova in the stool is negative. An eosinophilia often develops with the active disease, but since the eye involvement is usually late, eosinophilia is not often present.

There is no specific treatment. Systemic steroids often ameliorate the inflammatory response, but the best treatment is prevention. Children should be taught to wash their hands before eating. All dogs and cats should be dewormed.

In summary, choroiditis and chorioretinitis are serious eye diseases. In addition to the chorioretinal scar, which may be serious or benign depending on its position, many other complications may occur. Vitreous condensation may lead to severe visual reduction, and vitreous contraction may lead to retinal detachment. Glaucoma may develop from chronic inflammation in the anterior chamber. Macular edema, cataract, and total blindness with completely unresponsive electroretinogram, can all occur as a result of even low-grade long-standing chorioretinitis.

Treatment of chorioretinitis is often unsatisfactory even when a supposedly precise diagnosis has been made. Consequently, treatment is often pointed at controlling symptoms rather than the cause. Cycloplegics (atropine, Cyclogyl) and topical steroids are used to control the anterior effects of the disease. Systemic steroids and appropriate antibiotics are used to control the posterior disease. In all cases, the potential complications of the treatment must be balanced against the seriousness of the inflammation. Since these inflammations often last for years, it is often safe to accept a low level of chronic inflammation rather than continue high-dose steroid therapy.

RETINAL DEGENERATION

Retinal degenerations increase in incidence with age. There are two broad classifications: macular and peripheral. Peripheral degenerations are important in their relationship to retinal detachment.

MACULAR DEGENERATION

Senile macular degeneration encompasses a wide variation in ophthalmoscopic appearances. All seem to have a basic though variable progression. Most likely the underlying cause is an abnormality at the level of retinal pigment epithelium or at Bruch's membrane, the thin membrane between the pigment epithelium and choroid.

Breakdown of the Bruch's membrane is often signaled by drusen, which appear ophthalmoscopically to be oval yellow dots about the diameter of the major blood vessels. Histologically, they are mounds on Bruch's membrane. Pigment clumping at the macula usually occurs at this time. The next step is the development

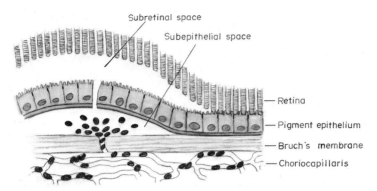

Figure 7-14. *Early macular degeneration demonstrating serous detachment of the retina and blood under the pigment epithelium. The blood may eventually seep under the retina.*

of abnormal fluid transfer through Bruch's membrane; this movement leads to elevation or a "blistering" of the retina inward—called *central serous retinopathy.* Fluorescein angiography at this time may demonstrate a point source of fluorescein pooling within the central serous blister, to indicate the site of abnormal fluid transfer. Treatment of this site with photocoagulation often stops the leakage and allows absorption of the blister.

Central serous retinopathy usually does not lead to the next step in the degenerative process, but it can. This next step may arise spontaneously, but is usually preceded by some visible disturbance of the macular pigment. For some unknown reason, an abnormal blood vessel from the choriocapillaris may grow through the defect in Bruch's membrane and lead to a subretinal hemorrhage, which will usually lead to a subretinal scar (Fig. 7-14). Unfortunately, the hemorrhage and subsequent scar almost always occur at the macula. Therefore, macular vision is affected immediately. Gradual progression over months or years occurs until the entire macula is destroyed.

The final appearance is that of a white subretinal scar mixed with pigment and a thinned and degenerated retina because of loss of normal nutrition (Fig. 7-15). The retina may be flat or elevated. The terms used are *disciform degeneration, Kuhnt-Junius, exudative* or *hemorrhagic maculopathy, senile macular degeneration,* and *involutional maculopathy.* All are names used for the same disease in different phases. The slow process of macular degeneration may take years to run its course. However, it is

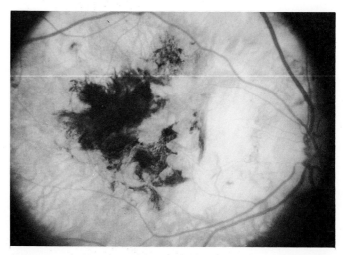

Figure 7-15. *Macular degeneration. Macula shows white sub-*
retinal scar mixed with dark pigment (Photo courtesy of
Frank Flanagin, Associated Retinal Consultants, Detroit.)

almost invariably bilateral, leading to severe reduction of central
vision.

MYOPIC DEGENERATION

Myopic degeneration occurs in patients who are very nearsighted.
The nearsighted eye is generally larger than normal and it is felt
that there is a mismatch between the size of the sclera and the
choroid and retina. This gives rise to a developmental stretching
and thinning of the choroid at the posterior pole. The ophthalmologic appearance is that of large, roughly oval, but irregular
white patches of absent choroid (Fig. 7-16). A dark spot at the
macula often signals the first episode of a steady downward
course. It is a deep hemorrhage and is called a Fuchs' spot. However, a great deal of atrophy may be present without central
visual loss, if the macula is spared. The most common site is the
posterior pole, and the retina is adversely affected by loss of the
normal nutrition to the rods and cones.

Nursing Care of Macular Degeneration

When a diagnosis of macular degenerative disease is made, the
patient's visual function is usually satisfactory. This vision con-

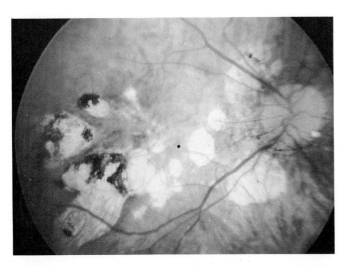

Figure 7-16. *Myopic degeneration. (Photo courtesy of Frank Flanagin, Associated Retinal Consultants, Detroit.)*

tinues for several years. However, the ultimate result of this disease is poor vision as the macula becomes destroyed. These degenerative conditions almost always become bilateral, causing severe limitations to even routine activity.

These patients are usually in the older age group, since a large percentage of macular degeneration is senile macular degeneration. Therefore they tend to be lonely. They are retired or near retirement, and their activities are limited to watching television, as reading becomes increasingly difficult. As vision continues to deteriorate, television viewing is no longer possible because of visual disability. These people are truly sensorily deprived. They become bored, lonely, and frightened as they lose sight and are forced to change some of their normal habits. A need for mobility training becomes apparent to the physician and nurse as sight decreases. The patient finds that while physically he can care for his own activities of daily living, he needs to learn the techniques of the blind or the visually handicapped. There is a need to teach the patient new homemaking methods—for example, how to conveniently set up the kitchen and use kitchen utensils and appliances. This training for the visually handicapped makes them able to manage their own activities of daily living.

Because the patients are older, their general health should be evaluated. Some patients may need supplemental vitamins because of poor dietary habits. The patient may find eating alone not so enjoyable and thus hesitates to take the time to cook, thus suffering from poor nutrition. Meals on Wheels may be a solution for these people; at least, they receive one cooked meal a day and may look forward to the conversation of the person delivering that meal—for some, the only daily social contact.

Trauma

Trauma may cause macular damage. The trauma must consist of a direct blow to the eye, although the lid may be closed at the time. Initially, the retina becomes edematous and has a grayish milky color. This edema invariably subsides, and the vision usually returns to normal. Occasionally, more serious damage may result in disruption of the choroid and pigment epithelium demonstrated by pigment clumping at the macula, and macular hemorrhage and reduced central vision. Not infrequently, following a severe blow, one or more narrow white crescents may be seen. This is characteristic of a choroidal rupture (Fig. 7–17). The curve of the crescent is always away from the disc, and the long axis is invariably vertical. The lesions may be nasal, temporal, or through the macula, but their presence almost always signals sufficient macular damage to cause reduced central vision.

Solar Burns

Another infrequent cause of macular trauma results from a solar burn. The result is a small area of pigment alteration and white scar in the center of the macula. This incident most commonly occurs when looking at an eclipse of the sun. It is extremely important to teach children the dangers of looking at an eclipse. In spite of community awareness, several eclipse burns usually occur within a major metropolitan area after an eclipse. Similar lesions have more recently been reported in young people who have been staring at the sun while under the influence of drugs (e.g., marijuana or LSD).

HEREDITARY INFLUENCES

Hereditary retinal degenerations do occur. Most of them have the eventual appearance of senile macular degeneration when they

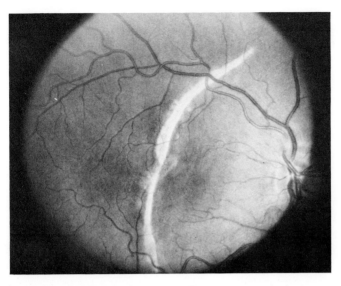

Figure 7-17. *Choroidal rupture. White crescent of sclera showing through the ruptured choroid on the temporal edge of the macula. (Photo courtesy of Frank Flanagin, Associated Retinal Consultants, Detroit.)*

have run their course. Their appearance at onset, progression, and inheritance are variable but often quite similar within a family. The final visual acuity may be very poor or rather good.

There is a group of hereditary pigmentary degenerations. The most common by far is *retinitis pigmentosa* (Fig. 7-18). It obtains its name from the classical appearance of retinal pigmentation in the form of bone spicules scattered initially in the midretinal periphery but later throughout most of the retina except the posterior pole. There is also narrowing of the retinal arteries and optic atrophy late in the disease. The initial symptom is usually night blindness, which may begin in early childhood; the retinal signs are often seen by the tenth year. The condition often progresses to total blindness by the age of 30. Peripheral field examination will demonstrate a scotoma in a ring around the midperiphery early in the disease. This gradually progresses centrally and peripherally, causing tunnel vision in the late stages of the disease.

There is no treatment for the disease. However, there is great variability in the course and final visual result. If the symptoms develop at an older age, the prognosis seems better.

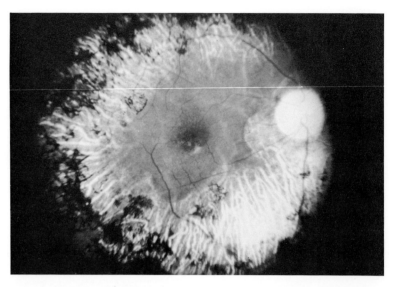

Figure 7-18. *Retinitis pigmentosa. Typical bone spicule pigmentation extends very close to macula in this photograph. Note atrophy of pigment layer and narrowing of retinal vessels. (Photo courtesy of Frank Flanagin, Associated Retinal Consultants, Detroit.)*

OPTIC NERVE

Degeneration of the optic nerve is signaled by a pale or white appearance of the optic disc. There are varying degrees of optic nerve degeneration (optic atrophy). The color of the optic disc varies from person to person, and the best method of distinguishing subtle changes is to compare the optic discs of the two eyes (Fig. 7-19). If the optic disc appears completely white, there is usually no light perception. The most common cause of optic atrophy is a previous optic neuritis. Multiple sclerosis, diabetes, systemic syphilis, and certain toxins such as methyl alcohol are the most common causes. Vascular occlusions of the vessels supplying the optic nerve may occur, either separately (rare), or in conjunction with an occlusion of the central retinal artery and cause optic atrophy. Trauma also may be a cause. The injury probably occurs either by contusion where the nerve courses through the bony optic canal or by fracture of the bony canal, causing direct compression of the nerve. Treatment, once atrophy has developed, is not effective.

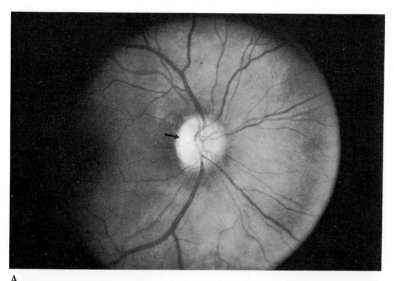

A

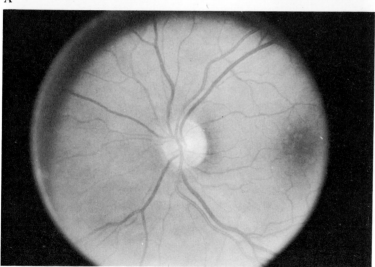

B

Figure 7–19. *Optic atrophy in same patient. A. Pallor of temporal portion of right optic nerve (arrow). B. Normal left optic nerve. (Photo courtesy of Frank Flanagin, Associated Retinal Consultants, Detroit.)*

Optic Neuritis

Inflammation of the optic nerve is called *optic neuritis.* It has been classically divided into *papillitis* if the inflammation is anterior and the disc is swollen, and *retrobulbar neuritis* if the inflammation is farther back in the nerve and the disc is not swollen.

The primary symptom is loss of vision. The vision may be severely reduced, for example, as low as light perception only, or it may be reduced only several lines on the eye chart. A visual field examination will demonstrate the extent of nerve involvement. In some cases only a small field deficiency (scotoma) will exist. This frequently is over the center of fixation.

Papillitis

Papillitis must be distinguished from papilledema and pseudopapilledema. The latter is a congenital condition in which the nerve has more glial tissue than normal at the disc and the disc is slightly elevated into the vitreous cavity. The vision is normal. Papilledema results from increased intracranial pressure (Fig. 7–20). It is usually bilateral, but rarely one eye may be affected before the other. The vision is usually not reduced in the early stages and the only abnormal finding (other than the appearance of the disc) may be an enlarged blind spot on the field exam. If papilledema is long standing, optic atrophy may develop and the vision will be affected. Brain tumor is the most common cause, and a thorough neurologic examination is always indicated. Papillitis always is associated with some visual loss, although the loss may not be proportionate to the ophthalmoscopic appearance. The disc is edematous and there are often exudates and hemorrhages. There may be tenderness over the globe, and pain in the orbit is common. A classical sign is pain on movement of the eye. The cause of papillitis is often difficult to ascertain. A thorough general physical examination should be performed with special attention to occult foci of infection such as teeth and tonsils. However, the results of even extensive evaluations are often disappointing and treatment must be empiric. Systemic steroids may be beneficial. They are usually used in high doses 120 to 160 mg/day for relatively short periods—days to weeks.

Retrobulbar Neuritis

Retrobulbar neuritis has signs and symptoms similar to papillitis, except that the disc appears ophthalmoscopically normal. The

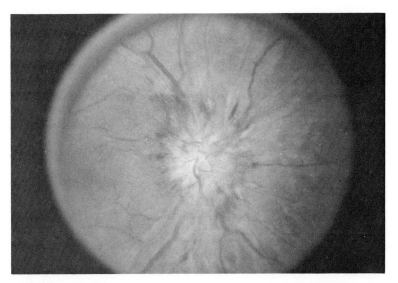

Figure 7-20. *Papilledema (edema of the optic disc). Note blurred appearance of disc margin and inability to see portions of major vessels on the disc caused by swelling of nerve tissue; dark linear spots indicate hemorrhages in the nerve fiber layer (so-called splinter hemorrhages). (Photo courtesy of Frank Flanagin, Associated Retinal Consultants, Detroit.)*

vision is reduced, but the field defect is small and usually involves the macula only, rarely extending beyond several disc diameters from the macula. The differential diagnosis is similar to that of papillitis but the most common cause is multiple sclerosis. Retrobulbar neuritis is particularly prone to recurrent episodes of inflammation and healing. The healing often occurs spontaneously, and the vision may return to normal between episodes. A classical late finding in retrobulbar neuritis is paleness of the temporal portion of the disc. This is particularly noticeable if the lesion is monocular. It is somewhat more difficult to evaluate if there has been binocular involvement. As with papillitis, the treatment is dependent upon the diagnosis. However, since the diagnosis is often obscure, systemic steroids are often used.

There are many toxic substances that will cause optic neuritis. Tobacco, particularly cigars, and alcohol ingestion may cause a central scotoma (more common in the presence of poor general nutrition). In addition, methyl alcohol poisoning is a serious threat both to vision and to life. Usually, even if the patient does recover, there is severe permanent visual loss. The treatment for all toxic optic neuritis is rapid diagnosis and the appropriate countermeasures, including removal of the toxic element and steroid therapy.

RETINAL ARTERY DISEASE

The central retinal artery, as it passes through the optic nerve, is identical to other arteries of equal size throughout the body. After its second branch within the retina, it loses its muscular coat, and the remainder of the visible retinal vessels are arterioles and venules. The vessel walls are normally transparent, and what is seen is actually the column of blood. The arteries have a more reddish-orange color and are narrower than the veins in a ratio of about 2:3.

The changes of aging described as arteriosclerosis consist of changes in transparency, changes in light reflex, and changes at the arteriolar-venous crossings. As the vessel walls thicken, the light reflex, which extends along the length of the vessel, becomes wider and brighter, eventually giving a burnished appearance to the vessel. Later as the vessel becomes more opaque, white lines show up along its sides and become larger until they meet, to obliterate the blood column from view. The other prominent changes occur at the arteriolar-venous crossing. The arterioles and venules are attached in a common adventitial sheath wherever they come together. Thus at the crossings, the venule is distorted as the arteriolar wall becomes thickened. This phenomenon is commonly referred to as *nicking* and is a result of a depression of the venule deeper into the retina as the arteriole thickens (Fig. 7–21).

Hypertensive changes are less easily noticed, and pure hypertensive changes rarely occur without previous existing arteriolosclerosis. The initial sign is that of narrowing of the arterioles—often patchy and usually transitory. Later, the bifurcations become more acute and hemorrhages (typically splinter hemorrhages rather than round or blot hemorrhages) and fluffy white exudates (soft exudates) appear. Later changes show marked retinal edema with the typical macular edema forming radiating lines in the shape of a star (macular star).

Treatment of these conditions should be directed toward the control of the systemic disease.

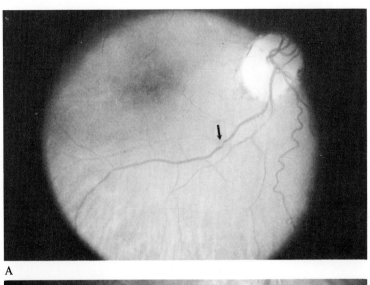

A

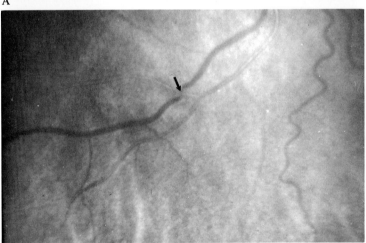

B

Figure 7-21. *Crossing changes. A. Crossing phenomenon (arrow). The vein is narrowed and distorted by arteriosclerotic artery. B. Close-up of crossing phenomenon seen in A. (Photo courtesy of Frank Flanagin, Associated Retinal Consultants, Detroit.)*

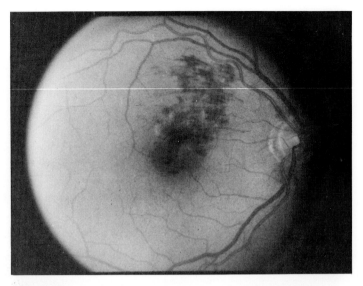

Figure 7-22. *Small branch retinal vein occlusion. Occluded vessel not apparent, but dark spots (hemorrhages) are in typical pattern. (Photo courtesy of Frank Flanagin, Associated Retinal Consultants, Detroit.)*

RETINAL VEIN OCCLUSION

Retinal vein occlusion is a sequela of the arteriosclerotic process. Occlusion may occur within the optic nerve, but most commonly at the level of the lamina cribrosa—a screenlike tissue at the outer level of sclera through which the optic nerve passes. Occlusion may also occur anywhere along the retinal veins but usually at a bifurcation. With occlusion, multiple, thick, irregularly oval retinal hemorrhages occur throughout the area drained by that vein (Fig. 7-22). In addition, retinal edema develops in the same area. If the macula is affected, central vision will suffer. If the macula is uninvolved, the central vision may remain normal but there will be decreased vision in the field involved. Vein occlusions may resolve spontaneously, and the retinal integrity may be restored.

Treatment consists of systemic anticoagulants. If macular edema persists, laser treatment may improve vision. There are two late complications of central retinal vein occlusions. Retinal or disc neovascularization may develop and lead to massive vitreous hemorrhage. Also, secondary glaucoma may develop.

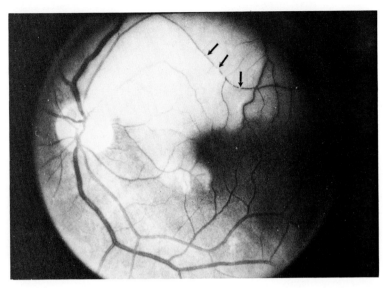

Figure 7-23. *Branch retinal artery occlusion. Note emboli in vessel (arrows). White area is area of retinal infarct and would look yellowish-white in fundus of eye. (Photo courtesy of Frank Flanagin, Associated Retinal Consultants, Detroit.)*

Retinal artery occlusions are much more serious. They may occur either due to arteriosclerotic changes or to emboli, and either central or branch occlusions may occur. The prognosis for visual return is poorer following an arterial occlusion because the blood supply to the inner retinal layers is stopped and an infarct occurs (Fig. 7-23). Clinically the retina has a yellowish, milky appearance and, if the macula is involved, the macular area stands out as a reddish dot within the yellowish retinal edema because the retinal tissue at the macula is thinner and does not become as edematous as the rest of the retina. Treatment is probably successful only if begun early, within hours. Emergency treatment should include exercise to increase blood pressure, and, if this fails, breathing in a paper bag to increase CO_2 content of the blood and thus dilate the blood vessels. In the very early stages of an arteriole occlusion symptomatic relief may occur rapidly. If these measures are unsuccessful, anticoagulants and vasodilators are used and surgical or medical attempts to lower the intraocular pressure should be employed. The prognosis is poor if the oc-

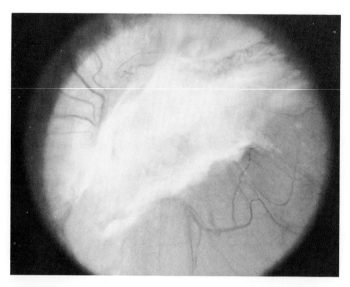

Figure 7–24. *Proliferative diabetic retinopathy. (Photo courtesy of Frank Flanagin, Associated Retinal Consultants, Detroit.)*

clusion has lasted for several hours. However, many times the clinical appearance is that of a total arterial occlusion, whereas fluorescein angiography demonstrates some blood flow. Therefore, treatment is indicated until the amount of retinal damage can be assessed. It is important to perform a thorough evaluation of the vascular system for anyone who has had a retinal occlusion. Particular attention should be paid to the carotid arteries where occlusive disease is often discovered.

DIABETIC RETINOPATHY

Diabetes has become a major retinal problem. With increasing longevity, more diabetic people are developing severe diabetic retinopathy. Diabetic retinopathy should be divided into two basic components: *nonproliferative* and *proliferative.* Proliferative retinopathy includes any neovascularization or fibrosis, whether elevated or on the surface of the retina (Fig. 7–24). Nonproliferative includes all other diabetic change, that is microaneurysms, blot hemorrhages, and retinal edema—particularly macular edema (Fig. 7–25). Proliferative retinopathy, in addition to neovascu-

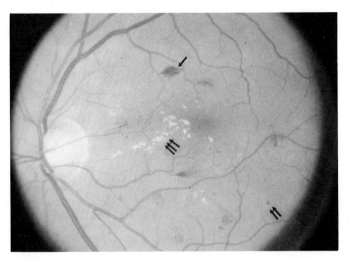

Figure 7–25. *Early diabetic (nonproliferative) retinopathy. (Single arrow points to blot hemorrhages; double arrow points to microaneurysm; triple arrow points to hard exudates.) (Photo courtesy of Frank Flanagin, Associated Retinal Consultants, Detroit.)*

larization or fibrosis or both, may be associated with vitreous hemorrhage, traction retinal detachment, and all the conditions present in the nonproliferative disease.

MEDICAL TREATMENT

Studies sponsored by the National Institute of Health have demonstrated that eyes with proliferative retinopathy do better when treated with the laser photocoagulator in a specific fashion (Fig. 7–26). The laser burns are placed in a pattern, one-half burn size apart, covering the area from the equator to the posterior pole, but sparing the area around the disc and macula (Fig. 7–27). Stereoscopic color photos of the posterior retina have been invaluable in evaluating the results of this treatment.

Nonproliferative retinopathy need not be treated except by maintenance of good diabetic control, unless macular edema develops. In this case, fluorescein angiography is often helpful in demonstrating retinal fluid leaks, which can be selectively treated by laser. The results of laser treatment for diabetic macular edema have been disappointing.

Unfortunately, even patients who have been under good diabetic

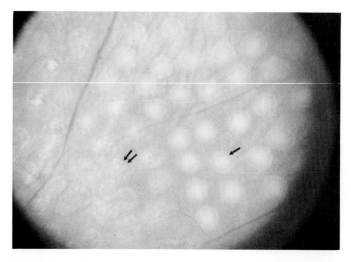

Figure 7-26. *Laser burns. Recent burns—within hours to days (single arrow); old burns—at least 10 days old (double arrow). (Photo courtesy of Frank Flanagin, Associated Retinal Consultants, Detroit.)*

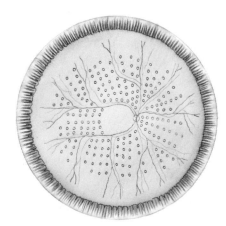

Figure 7-27. *Diabetic retinopathy, laser scatter pattern. Small circles indicate laser scars.*

control often develop proliferative disease and its complications after many years. Most experts feel that the person who has been dependent on insulin for 20 years probably will have some proliferative disease even if control has been good. Photocoagulation does not always stop progression of the disease, and vitrectomy has, therefore, become essential in managing later complications. Vitrectomy has been proved to be very effective in removing vitreous hemorrhage and in severing vitreoretinal membranes. These membranes form a scaffold on which neovascular tissue grows and also cause traction retinal detachment. Removal of these membranes will often lead to reattachment of a traction retinal detachment. Also, neovascular and proliferative tissue tends to shrink when the tense membranous scaffold is eliminated.

NURSING CARE

The patients who have diabetic retinopathy need expert nursing care. They need emotional and physical care because of their diabetic retinopathy, but also need assessment of their knowledge of diabetes and reinforcement or teaching for their chronic disease—diabetes. We have found that patients generally possess the basic knowledge for giving themselves good maintenance care. However, there are some who have a very limited knowledge base and need much basic instruction. To give total patient care then, the nurse must reassess the need for teaching care of the diabetic. Many hospitals have quality-assurance programs that are noteworthy. The following questionnaire, utilized at Evanston Hospital, seems to give a good indication of where to reinforce and where to teach concepts of care that are not understood by the patient.

Diabetes Questionnaire*

1. Date of onset (How long have you had diabetes?) _____
2. What happens in diabetes? _____
   _____
3. Medication for diabetes—Oral (kind) _____
   Insulin (How does it act?) _____
   a. Do you give your own insulin? _____
   b. How? (Kind-Amount-Strength-Time-Type of Syringe) _____
   _____
   c. Where? (Sites-Rotation) _____
   d. Do you make adjustments in your insulin? _____
   e. What if you are too ill to eat? What do you do? _____
   _____
4. Urine Testing
   a. Do you test your urine? _____

*From Rita Garber, R.N. and June Werner, R.N., Evanston Hospital, Evanston, IL. Used with permission.

    b. What kind of test do you use?_____

    c. What times during the day do you test? _____

    _____

    d. Do you keep a record? _____

    e. Do you test for acetone? (When?) _____

    f. What does acetone mean to you? _____

5. Diet

    a. Why do people with diabetes need to be careful about what they eat?_____

    b. Do you eat mostly at home or out? _____

    c. What times? _____

    d. Do you ever skip meals or make a change in the time you eat? (Reasons) _____

    e. Have you ever been given a diet plan and are you able to follow it well? _____

    f. Who prepares meals? (Weighed and Measured) _____

6. Insulin reactions

    a. Have you ever had a reaction? _____

    b. What usually happens to you? _____

    _____

    c. What do you do for it? _____

    d. Who at home can give you insulin if necessary? _____

7. Do you carry diabetic identification? (What type?) _____

8. Acidosis

    a. Are you familiar with the word *acidosis*? If so, what happens and what do you do? _____

    _____

9. Do you cut your toenails? _____ How? _____

10. What is your usual daily activity? _____

    _____

11. Do people at home or work know what to do if you have signs of an insulin reaction or signs of acidosis? _____

12. Do you have any special difficulties? _____

    _____

    _____

13. Is there any area of diabetic management that you feel you need more instruction in? _____

    _____

Name _____ Birthdate _____

Address _____ Occupation _____

Relatives with diabetes _____

For the diabetic to learn to live with the disease and to comply to a relatively set regimen, some knowledge of pathophysiology is necessary. The basic concept of diabetes must be understood for a patient to comply with a therapeutic regimen. The patient needs to know that diabetes occurs when there is an insufficient amount of insulin found in the islets of Langerhans of the pancreas. This insufficiency causes a dysfunction in the metabolism of carbohydrates, because insulin plays a major role in metabolism. Because of this insufficient insulin there is a dysfunction of metabolism. The patient develops the primary symptoms of diabetes polyuria, polydipsia, and polyphagia.

From such a simple explanation, the basic concepts of therapeutic treatment or maintenance can be discussed. The need for insulin or an oral hypoglycemic agent can be reiterated. The nurse may stress the kind of insulin the patient is receiving, the technique of giving one's own injection as well as the sites and importance of rotating sites of injection. Because patients with diabetic retinopathy have possibly had several hemorrhages previously and lost some vision, they may already be using some techniques and aids for the visually handicapped. Since maintaining a relatively constant blood glucose level is desirable, the patient needs to receive his correct dosage of insulin at the prescribed time. There are various types of aids available to assist patients in being self-sufficient in their own care. (See Appendix I.)

The patient who is in the hospital for diabetic retinopathy may be in a period of fluctuating vision and may leave the hospital with substantially less vision than on admission. Nurses should then be aware of the possibility of needing an aid for maintaining accuracy in insulin administration.

Methods of testing urine should also be reevaluated since sight is impaired. Since all of these tests require color discrimination, the patient may no longer be able to do this for himself. A family member or a close friend may do this. The other person should be nearby, because if urine stands for periods of time, it will begin to decompose and thus give an inaccurate reading. Judgment and planning on the part of the nurse as to feasibility of urine testing is helpful to the continuation of the self-care procedure. The American Foundation for the Blind is currently developing an electronic urine tester.

Frequently, patients with diabetic retinopathy will have guilt feelings as well as some depression over their vision impairment. The patient may feel he has not been complying as he should to his diet and therapeutic regimen. Indeed, most patients deviate at some time from their diets. Even the slightest deviation can be "haunting" the patient. Many theories exist as to the progression of retinopathy; most patients who have been insulin dependent for 20 years or more will usually have moderately advanced diabetic retinopathy. It is felt that even patients who have complied with treatment may suffer severe diabetic retinal disease and visual loss because of long duration of the disease. A common misconception held by nurses is that the disease progresses only because of noncompliance to a therapeutic regimen. Certainly, any patient with proliferative diabetic retinopathy can worsen even though the glucose level is strictly controlled.

Our belief is that reinforcement of diet is essential. In a hospital setting, the clinical dietitian can give new ideas and new insights into creative meal planning. For some patients, this may be necessary; for others it will be reinforcement. A source of consolation and encouragement to the compliant patient is the realization that even by following an acceptable regimen, there is a "normal progression" of the chronic disease.

The complications of hypoglycemia, hyperglycemia, and circulatory impairment should also be reinforced. Table 7–1 is a teaching plan that has proved helpful in giving some ideas as to a systematic manner of presenting instructions to patients, or initiating an effective clinical teaching program and environment.

DISEASES AFFECTING THE RETINA

TOXEMIA OF PREGNANCY

Toxemia of pregnancy may affect the retina, causing constriction of the retinal arterial tree. This phenomenon occurs only in the presence of hypertension. The constriction may affect only one or two branches, may be very patchy in its distribution, or may be widespread, constricting all vessels. In the more advanced stages, retinal hemorrhages and exudates occur. Termination of the pregnancy invariably reverses the abnormal process. Occasionally, following more severe exudative changes, sclerosis of the retinal vessels and disruption of the retinal pigment epithelium may persist. Less frequently, permanent visual reduction may remain. Occasionally, retinal detachment will develop secondary to abnormal fluid accumulation under the retina.

Table 7-1. *Patient Care Plan—Education for the Diabetic Patient**

Teaching Plan	Teaching Process	Learning Evaluation

Urine testing
Teaching completed
by _____
date _____
	Types of urine testing
	  Keto-Diastix
	  Diastix
	  Ketostix
	  Tes-Tape
	  Clinitest and Acetest
	  All are available and acceptable, assess which would be best for patient to use after discharge, and teach
	Methods of collection of urine specimen
	  Long specimen—Empty bladder completely
	  Short specimen—Collect urine specimen 30 min after discarding long specimen
	  Time of day—Before meals and at bedtime unless otherwise ordered
	  If container is used for the collection of the specimen, be sure it is clean
	  Brittle and juvenile diabetics should keep a written daily record of urine testing results; all others are encouraged to do so.
		Correct return demonstration and interpretation by
		☐ Patient
		☐ Family or significant other
		_____
		_____
		_____
		Comments: _____
		_____
		_____
		_____
		_____
		_____

Pathophysiology of diabetes mellitus
Teaching completed
by _____
date _____
	The Pancreas
	  Location
	  Function
	    Normal
	    Abnormal
	  Teaching aids available:
	  Audiovisual "Getting Started" *Beginning* (cassette tape & booklet)
		Correct interpretation and return of information by
		☐ Patient
		☐ Family or significant other
		Literature given to patient: _____
		_____
		_____

continued

*From June Werner, R.N. Copyright © 1976 by Evanston Hospital, Evanston, IL. Used with permission.

Table 7-1. (Continued)

Teaching Plan	Teaching Process	Learning Evaluation

	Audiovisual "What Is Diabetes" *Intermediate* (16 mm film)
	Book, *How to Live with Diabetes* by Dolger and Seeman, pp. 18–21. *Advanced*
	Potential contributing factors
	  Obesity
	  Family history
	  Age
	  Surgical intervention
	  Drug induced
	  Viral theory (Refer to *How to Live with Diabetes* by Dolger and Seeman, pp. 21–28)
		Audiovisual aids used: _____
		_____
		_____
		Comments: _____
		_____
		_____
		_____

Insulin administration
Teaching completed
by _____
date _____
	Insulin
	  Types of insulin
	  Long, intermediate, and short acting
	  Mixture of pork and beef, beef, or pork
	  Storage, travel, and expiration date
	  Available strengths
	Sites of injection
	Rotation
	  Possible areas for injection
	  Rotation of sites using the calendar method
	  Inspection of skin
	Assemble equipment for patient injection (label all equipment to be left at bedside for practice only, *NOT STERILE*)
	  Cotton balls, small container, 70% isopropyl alcohol
	  Syringe, needle, insulin, rotation schedule
	  Orange or tissue-test material
	Injection technique
	  Single insulin administration
		Correct return explanation of action, peak time and duration of the type of insulin to be used by the patient by
		  ☐ Patient
		  ☐ Family or significant other
		Comments: _____
		_____
		_____
		_____

Mixing insulins (be aware of attending physician's preference as
  to whether insulin can be mixed or *injected separately*)
Use of glucagon
Explanation and demonstration of injection
Practice by patient
Patient administers insulin

Correct return explanation and
demonstration by
☐ Patient
☐ Family or significant other
☐ Rotation
☐ Skin inspection
☐ Assembling equipment
☐ Administration of insulin
Comments: _____

Hyperglycemia and
hypoglycemia
Teaching completed
by _____
date _____

Hyperglycemia—elevation of blood glucose above normal. Signs and
symptoms include
Excessive thirst (polydipsia)
Frequent urination (polyuria)
Extreme hunger (polyphagia)
Fatigue and lethargy
Visual disturbances, blurring of vision
Weight loss
Skin disorders such as boils, infection, itching
Uncontrolled, prolonged hyperglycemia leads to acidosis or diabetic
ketoacidosis; signs and symptoms include
Dry, flushed skin
Acetone, fruity breath
Kussmaul's respiration, rapid breathing
Sunken, soft eyeballs
Fever, dehydration, nausea, and vomiting
Abdominal cramping
Tachycardia, rapid pulse
Decreased level of consciousness
Unconsciousness
Hypoglycemia—abnormally low, or rapid, extreme drop in blood
glucose level; signs and symptoms include
Mild hunger is a very early sign

Correct return explanation of
☐ Hyperglycemia
☐ Acidosis
☐ Hypoglycemia
by
☐ Patient
☐ Family or significant other
Comments: _____

continued

Table 7-1. (Continued)

Teaching Plan	Teaching Process	Learning Evaluation
	Sweating Dizziness Palpitation } Early signs Pale, moist skin Shallow breathing Trembling Blurred or double vision } Late signs Mental confusion and disorientation Very strange behavior Loss of consciousness	Correct return demonstration and interpretation by ☐ Patient ☐ Family or significant others of ☐ General skin care ☐ Foot care ☐ Exercise and employment ☐ Identification ☐ Sick-day guidelines Comments: _____

Activities of daily living
Teaching completed by ____
date ____
	Skin care (general)
	Bathe daily with good perineal hygiene, dry well
	Avoid tight fitting clothing
	Avoid skin exposure to temperature extremes
	  Hot water bottles
	  Heating pads
	  Frostbite
	Avoid irritants such as chemicals, dyes, bleaches, or detergents
	Use extreme caution to avoid cuts (i.e., shaving), bruises, fractures, and report any signs of infection to physician
	If skin is dry use appropriate lotions or oils
	Foot care
	Wash and dry feet well daily
	Inspect feet daily
	  Between toes
	  Dorsal surface
	Inspect entire extremity from toes to knees
	Use mirror if necessary to visualize all areas	

continued

Proper fitting shoes, socks, stockings

No bare feet

Change socks daily (no darns or seams)

Toenail care

Cut nails straight across

If nails thickened or unable to cut, seek professional care by physician or designated podiatrist

If corns, calluses, or bunions are present, don't cut

May use emery board or pumice stone gently

Don't use any commercial preparations

Ask physician for appropriate referral if surgical or medical intervention is necessary

Use lambs wool (not cotton balls) to keep toe surfaces separated whenever necessary

Employment and exercise

Employment or school

Let employer or teacher and health service know you are a diabetic

Don't skip meals, follow mealtime patterns

Wear necessary identification

Carry at least 10 gm of glucose or fast-acting CHO

Recreational activity

Desired physical activity may be participated in and pursued without limitation if diet and insulin are adjusted accordingly

If more activity than usual will be engaged in, check with doctor about changes in insulin and diet requirements

Travel

Travel

There are no travel restrictions anywhere in the world

Take into consideration the cuisine of the country and determine if diet requirements can be easily met

Be aware of the various time changes and that these may affect meal times.

Table 7-1. (Continued)

Teaching Plan	Teaching Process	Learning Evaluation
	Know how to say, "I am a diabetic, get me to a doctor, or give me candy or orange juice," in the various languages of the countries you are visiting	
	Carry urine testing equipment	
Identification	Identification	
	Always wear identification tag and card such as Medic-Alert	
	In wallet or purse carry name of doctor, insulin dosage, diet, and other pertinent medical facts	
Sick day guide-lines	Illness	
	Never skip a dose of insulin	
	If nauseated, take sips of ginger ale or cola syrup (use regular nondietetic variety)	
	Test urine frequently, test for ketones	
	Call doctor immediately upon feeling ill	
Follow-up care	Suggested doctor care	
	See attending physician every three months or whenever necessary	
	See dentist regularly. Be sure to tell him that you are a diabetic	
	Women should see gynecologist twice a year	
	Eye examination by ophthalmologist twice a year	
	Annual chest x-ray	
	Health care agencies	
	VNA	
	Public health nurse	
	American Diabetes Association	
	Meals on Wheels	
	Homemakers	
	FISH	

Diet instruction
Teaching completed
by _____
date _____

Hospital discharge planner
Hospital diabetic dietician
Diet instruction
  To be done by diabetic dietician
  Student teacher should be observed by dietician
  Diabetic dietician should be notified as soon as possible of all new and old diabetic admissions
  Dietician will assist old diabetics as needed or by referral
  When old diabetic is readmitted, check to see if patient has diet file
Instruction on basic food exchanges
Diet adjustments for
  Personal preference
  Ethnic or religious restrictions
  Use of alcohol
  Dietary compensation for increased exercise

Correct return demonstration of selecting diet and interpretation of food exchanges by
☐ Patient
☐ Family or significant other
☐ Explanation of basic food exchange
☐ Able to correctly choose diet for 3 meals
List booklets given to patient:
_____
_____

Comments: _____
_____
_____

SICKLE CELL DISEASE

Retinal abnormalities are frequently found in patients with sickle cell (SC) disease. Persons afflicted by sickle cell disease demonstrate sickle shaped red blood cells in the presence of reduced oxygen. These blood cells mechanically do not negotiate small blood vessels readily and cause microvascular obstructions. The sickling phenomenon results from abnormal hemoglobin. Electrophoresis has been able to demonstrate over 20 hemoglobin variants, which have been labeled by letters: e.g., normal adult (A), sickle (S). The others have been labeled C, D, E and so on. The person who has one normal (A) and one abnormal (S) gene is said to have the trait and usually does not show signs of the disease. If a person has two abnormal genes (SS, SC, CC), he has sickle cell disease and will manifest the abnormal symptoms in varying degrees. There is a high racial predilection to the abnormal hemoglobin diseases. In this country the majority of those affected are members of the black race.

The retinal abnormalities are a result of vascular thrombosis. In sickle cell disease, it is not uncommon to find vascular narrowing, tortuosity, and obliteration of vessels, which may lead to hemorrhages and proliferation of fibrotic and neovascular tissue. SC disease has a high incidence of retinal abnormalities causing obstruction of the arteries and veins. Patchy areas of empty capillaries can be demonstrated on fluorescein angiography. These areas are usually in the midperiphery. They lead to preretinal fibrosis, distortion of the vessels in the local area, and the development of arteriovenous anastomosis. Often a patch of these vessels is elevated by preretinal fibrous traction, causing the vessels to form the shape of a fan. This has been called a *sea-fan.* It is characteristic of sickle cell disease and often leads to severe vitreous hemorrhage.

Photocoagulation of the abnormal vascular tissue is the most effective treatment. Patients require frequent evaluation to identify newly formed abnormal areas before they lead to serious complications.

TUMORS

BENIGN

Most intraocular tumors are choroidal. The most common intraocular tumor by far is the benign choroidal nevus. Nevi appear as roughly oval flat lesions that are brown, gray, or black (Fig. 7-28).

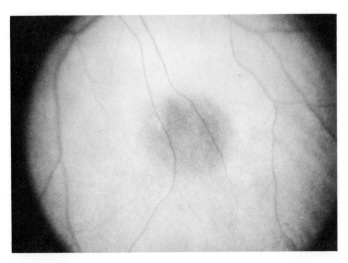

Figure 7–28. *Choroidal nevus. Flat pigmented lesion that stands out in choroid. (Photo courtesy of Frank Flanagin, Associated Retinal Consultants, Detroit.)*

They are rarely larger than 2 disc diameters in size. The retinal blood vessels run over the lesion. Nevi do not affect vision and the major concern is to differentiate them from malignant melanomas. Melanomas are elevated and increase in size. They also pick up fluorescein dye on angiography. Nevi do none of these.

Choroidal hemangiomas are difficult to diagnose clinically. They are not pigmented, and, when they are seen clinically, they give a subtle yellowish-red appearance to the normal choroidal pattern. Hemangiomas frequently cause fluid leakage under the retina with either localized or massive regional detachment. The diagnosis is made by fluorescein angiography. Treatment consists of trans-scleral cryothermy application or photocoagulation.

MALIGNANT

Choroidal Melanoma

Malignant melanoma of the choroid is the most common malignant tumor found in the eye. The characteristics are extremely variable. The melanoma is always elevated but may appear mound-like (Fig. 7–29) or may be highly elevated and even globular on a narrow stalk. The color varies from dark brown to yellowish-

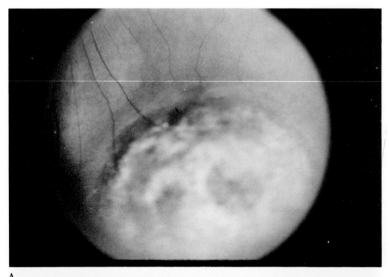

A

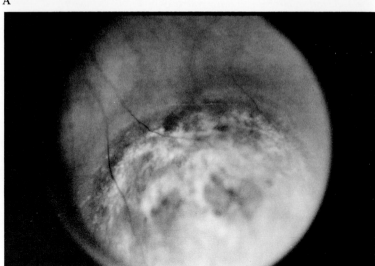

B

Figure 7-29. *A. Elevated intraocular tumor. Focus is on surface of retina. Note retinal vessels are in focus. B. Elevated intraocular tumor focused on surface of tumor. Note retinal vessels are out of focus. This view is focused on surface of tumor. (Photo courtesy of Frank Flanagin, Associated Retinal Consultants, Detroit.)*

white (amelanotic). There is usually an associated retinal detachment, and often subretinal hemorrhage. Fluorescein angiography will demonstrate intensive hyperfluorescence of the lesion. A more recently used test is the phosphorus 32 radioactive isotope uptake test. Phosphorus is given orally or intravenously, and the uptake in the lesion is counted by means of a special Geiger counter 48 to 72 hours later. If the count over the lesion is approximately double that of a control area, the lesion is considered malignant. If the lesion is anterior, the count can be taken through the conjunctiva. If, however, the lesion is posterior, a conjunctival incision must be made to apply the counter directly over the lesion. Ultrasonography can be used to document an elevated lesion as well as ascertain the density of the lesion. Ultrasonography has become indispensable in evaluating the posterior globe when corneal scar or cataract obscures ophthalmoscopic evaluation. Frequently, unsuspected tumors are discovered.

Choroidal melanomas do not have the same grave prognosis as do melanomas of the skin. Survival is influenced greatly by the cell type. In lesions with the most malignant cell type (epithelioid), the ten-year survival is about 20 percent. In lesions with the least malignant cell type (spindle), the ten-year survival may reach 80 percent.

Treatment of most large melanomas requires enucleation of the eye. Small lesions can be destroyed by radiation (cobalt plaques sutured on the sclera over the lesion for days to weeks), photocoagulation, diathermy, and cryothermy. Although enucleation is the safest form of treatment, metastases may often become evident months or years after the eye has been enucleated.

Metastases

Metastatic choroidal tumors are not common. When they occur, the most frequent site of origin is the breast (about 60 percent of all metastatic tumors to the choroid), with the only other large group arising in the lung. Metastatic carcinomas have been documented from most organs. Lymphomas also may develop choroidal metastases.

Metastatic lesions are usually situated in the posterior pole because the major choroidal arteries enter the globe there. These lesions may be multiple, are usually unpigmented (otherwise differentiation is difficult), and often cause retinal detachments. A thorough general evaluation almost invariably demonstrates the primary site.

Treatment should be directed toward the primary lesion. However, many metastases are radiosensitive, and x-ray therapy will often cause rapid destruction of the metastasis and absorption of the retinal detachment.

Retinoblastoma

Retinoblastoma is the only malignant retinal tumor of consequence in both number and severity. Early studies indicated an incidence of about 0.003 percent of live births. With better diagnostic methods and better treatment techniques, however, many of these patients are surviving to have children. The incidence is, therefore, expected to increase. Retinoblastoma is a disease of childhood. Most retinoblastomas are discovered by the age of two years and it is rare to diagnose a case in a child older than 5 years. There is no sexual prevalence. In about 60 percent of cases, retinoblastoma is first seen as a white pupil or "cat's eye" (Fig. 7–30A). This must be differentiated from several other conditions, among which are cataract, endophthalmitis, and retrolental fibroplasia. The other common signs are crossed eyes, poor vision, or inflamed eye.

Clinically, the lesion appears as a white or creamy white well-defined mound of variable height, size, and shape. It is usually round or oval, but there may be multiple lesions of various size, and they may be confluent. Seeding, small round lesions on the surface of the retina or in the vitreous, and chalky white or pearly patches on the surface of the larger lesions are considered to be almost pathognomonic (Fig. 7–30B). The chalky appearance is the result of necrosis within the tumor. This is often demonstrable on x-ray.

The tumor spreads by direct extension into the optic nerve. It then gains access to the cranial cavity through the subarachnoid space, so that metastasis to the brain and skull occur early. Metastases by lymphatics and bloodstream eventually spread to the bones of the skull, the long bones, and the viscera.

Heredity is an important topic in counseling parents of children with this tragic disease. Most authorities agree that 96 percent of cases are sporadic in nature and do not involve a hereditary condition. The chances of retinoblastoma occurring in a sibling of a sporadic case is less than 4 percent. However, if another case has occurred in the family, the risk then becomes approximately

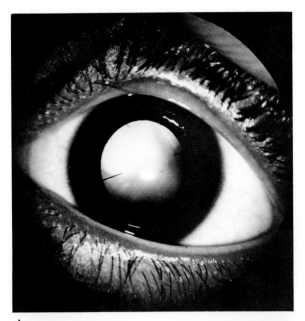

A

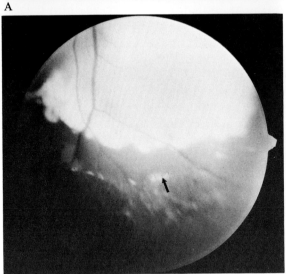

B

Figure 7-30. *Retinoblastoma. A. White pupillary reflex. The so-called cat's eye reflex. B. Fundus picture of edge of large retinoblastoma lesion. Arrow points to one of several "seeds" of tumor adjacent to major lesion. (Photo courtesy of Frank Flanagin, Associated Retinal Consultants, Detroit.)*

40 percent. By the same token, a patient with a healed unilateral tumor and no hereditary history has only a 5 to 10 percent chance of producing a child with retinoblastoma. If, however, an affected child is produced, the parent must be considered to have had a hereditary lesion, and the risk for additional children becomes 40 percent. A parent who has had bilateral disease has a very great chance of having a hereditary trait, even in the absence of a family history, and the risk to offspring would be 40 percent.

Treatment of unilateral disease is enucleation. Conscious effort should be made to remove as much of the optic nerve as possible, since the tumor often invades the nerve. If both eyes are involved, the less involved eye can be treated by photocoagulation, cryothermy applied to the scleral surface at the tumor site, radiation, and chemotherapy, separately or in combination.

RETINAL DETACHMENT

Retinal detachment is the condition in which the sensory retina separates from the pigment epithelium and collapses into the vitreous cavity. There is no pain. The primary symptom is loss of vision, and the visual loss depends on the amount of retina that detaches. Detachment usually begins in the periphery and spreads circumferentially and posteriorly. Thus, one quadrant of the retina may be detached, causing loss of vision in one quadrant of the visual field. If the detachment spreads to involve the macula, the visual acuity may become very poor, even causing inability to see the chart. However, a large detachment may be present in the periphery without involving the macula, and the visual acuity would remain normal. The tendency is for detachments to enlarge until all the retina is detached. The only remaining areas of attachment to the wall of the eye will be at the ora serrata and at the optic disc.

Retinal detachments should be classified into two categories: *rhegmatogenous,* from the Greek *rhegma* (rupture) and nonrhegmatogenous, or secondary.

NONRHEGMATOGENOUS

Nonrhegmatogenous detachments may be subdivided into traction and exudative. In either case, retinal holes are not the cause of the detachment, although they may occur from degenerative changes in a previously existing detachment. Traction detachments,

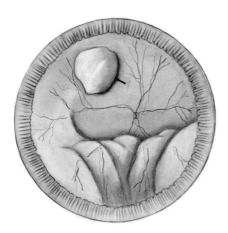

Figure 7–31. *Nonrhegmatogenous retinal detachment. Solid tumor (arrow) is above. The detachment is most prominent below.*

as the name implies, develop due to development of fibrotic membranes within the vitreous. These membranes frequently develop attachments to the retina, and, as they contract, they pull the retina away from its normal position. These membranes develop as a result of intraocular inflammation, perforation of the globe, and vitreous hemorrhage. Fibrotic membranes are particularly common in diabetic and sickle cell retinopathy, which are associated with abnormal retinal vessels and vitreous hemorrhage.

Exudative detachments are secondary to intraocular inflammation, intraocular tumors, or certain systemic diseases. Usually the inflammation is nonspecific, and a thorough physical examination, including laboratory studies, is unproductive. Occasionally, a specific uveitis or chorioretinitis can be identified. Malignant melanomas and metastatic tumors are two of the intraocular tumors commonly associated with detachment (Fig. 7–31). Toxemia of pregnancy, certain kidney diseases, and certain blood dyscrasias may also cause exudative detachment.

Treatment of nonrhegmatogenous detachment depends on treatment of the cause. Traction retinal detachments frequently can be resolved by vitrectomy. (See Chap. 6, Surgery, p. 140.) Once the membranes are removed, the retina will settle into its normal position. Detachments secondary to inflammation usually require corticosteroid therapy, often systemic, in addition to

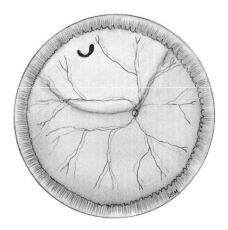

Figure 7–32. *Superior temporal retinal detachment with a horseshoe tear, anterior to the equator at 11 o'clock.*

specific therapy if a cause can be discovered. If a tumor is present, eradication of the tumor is essential. Most systemic diseases are readily identified and, if the disease can be controlled, the detachment improves rapidly.

RHEGMATOGENOUS

Rhegmatogenous detachments are caused by hole formation in the sensory retina (Fig. 7–32). Fluid from the vitreous cavity seeps through the hole and separates the sensory retina from the pigment epithelium. The holes are caused by degenerative change in the vitreous, the retina, or both. Although minor trauma may precipitate retinal hole formation in the presence of already existing retinal degeneration, severe and usually direct trauma to the eye, such as a blow with a fist, is necessary to cause a retinal hole in a healthy retina.

RETINAL HOLES

Usually, vitreous degeneration and collapse of the vitreous body is the primary precursor of retinal hole formation. In the young, the vitreous is a solid gel in direct contact with and with attachments to the retina. By middle age, the vitreous begins to contract and eventually it collapses into the anterior portion of the vitreous cavity with attachments at and anterior to the equator. The trac-

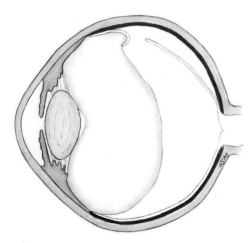

Figure 7-33. *Posterior vitreous detachment with adhesion of vitreous to the anterior edge of a retinal tear and detachment of the retina.*

tion at the sites of attachment in some people eventually leads to retinal degeneration and then hole formation (Fig. 7-33).

Retinal holes do not necessarily lead to retinal detachment. Continued vitreous traction at the hole site is certainly the major precipitating factor in the development of retinal detachment. If the vitreous separates from around the hole, the hole may remain for years without leading to a detachment. However, continued traction may cause immediate progression to a retinal detachment. Minor trauma in the presence of a retinal hole may lead to retinal detachment.

These pathologic vitreous changes cause two other prominent symptoms associated with rhegmatogenous retinal detachments: light flashes and floaters. Light flashes are caused by vitreous traction on the retina. Since the retina has only sensory nerve components, it can respond in only one way when stimulated. Thus, this stimulation causes a sensation of light. The flashes are usually described as being like heat lightning. They are subtle and usually seen on arising in the morning or entering a darkened room.

Floaters are the result of thickened particles within the vitreous cavity. Most commonly, they are caused by thickened vitreous clumps or by vitreous hemorrhage, which often occurs as a retinal hole forms and tears across a retinal blood vessel. Vitreous hemorrhage may assume almost any configuration but is most often described as a web, clumps, or spots. They float back and forth in the vitreous fluid, thus the term *floaters.*

The onset of flashes or floaters demands thorough examination of the retina, including examination of the peripheral retina. Vitreous hemorrhage may be a result of a momentary blood vessel leak secondary to vitreous traction. Floaters may be the result of vitreous shrinkage only. Light flashes may indicate vitreoretinal traction without hole formation. But these symptoms may result from early stages of serious retinal disease. Treatment requires observation and patience. Spontaneous resolution is the rule, although floaters may remain for months or years. Repeat observation in the presence of persistent symptoms is necessary, to discover progressive retinal changes should they occur.

Retinal holes almost always form in the periphery, near or anterior to the equator. Therefore, retinal detachments will begin in the periphery. Their progression to total detachment may be very slow or almost instantaneous. If progression is slow, the patient may notice a dark shadow of blurred or absent vision progress from one quadrant of the visual field toward the center of vision, and then involve the entire field of vision. The vision in any area of attached retina will remain normal. After the entire retina detaches, the vision is rarely better than count fingers, and often poorer.

TREATMENT

The treatment for retinal holes and retinal detachments is basically the same, that is, to cause a scar to develop around the hole between the retina and the choroid. The techniques vary depending on whether a detachment is present, where the hole is located, and preference of the surgeon.

Three modalities are commonly used to form the scar: photocoagulation, diathermy, and cryothermy. Photocoagulation requires a special instrument incorporating a strong light source and an ophthalmoscopic delivery system capable of focusing a small dot of light on the retina. Several designs are available. They use either a xenon light source or one of several laser sources, the most widely used being the argon laser. An observation light is directed through the dilated pupil, and by ophthalmoscopic control the surgeon focuses this light on the retinal hole. Release of a shutter applies a momentary burst of the light resulting in a burn to the retina and choroid. The diameter of the burn can be varied from about 0.05 mm to 1.0 mm. The lasers will produce an equal burn with less energy output than the xenon light source. The additional energy given off by the xenon light causes excessive heat buildup, and the patient will experience pain if an anesthetic is not injected behind the eye (retrobulbar anesthesia). Most people tolerate the minor discomfort of laser application without a retrobulbar injection. Diathermy and cryothermy are both applied to the surface of the sclera. Diathermy causes a heat burn. Cryothermy causes a freeze. The choice of modality often depends on the position of the retinal hole. If it is posterior, photocoagulation is easier, since cryothermy or diathermy would require a conjunctival incision. If it is anterior, the pupil may not dilate enough for focusing of the photocoagulator.

The effect of each of these methods is to cause a choroiditis. If the retina is in contact with the choroid, a chorioretinitis will develop and, as it heals, will leave a chorioretinal scar that will surround the retinal hole and effectively obliterate it. If the retina is not detached, this scar should suffice.

If the retina is detached, a second step must be added. Something must be done to approximate the retina and choroid. This can be achieved by draining the fluid (subretinal fluid) by making a drainage hole through the sclera and choroid, by indenting the globe under the hole, or by doing both. Indenting or inbuckling the globe is favored by most retinal surgeons because, in addition to apposing the retina and choroid, this technique will reduce vitreous traction on the retina. This operation has been named *scleral buckle.*

The first step in performing a scleral buckle is to incise the conjunctiva and expose the sclera. The four rectus muscles are usually isolated and tagged with a suture. These sutures are used to rotate the eye so that the equator can be viewed. The retina is then examined with the indirect ophthalmoscope and a mark placed on the sclera at the site of each retinal hole (Fig. 7–34). The implant is indented at the hole site either by placing mattress sutures (Fig. 7–35) so they will indent it (explant) or by dissecting partial-thickness flaps of sclera, which are then sewn over the implant (Fig. 7–36). The sutures indenting the implant are not tied until the eye is softened by draining the subretinal (detachment) fluid (Fig. 7–37). In some instances, if the detachment is low enough and the globe soft enough, the implant can be indented to bring the choroid in contact with the retina without

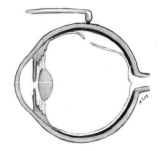

Figure 7–34. *Localization of retinal hole in detached retina by depressing sclera with a diathermy probe. Site of hole is marked on the surface of the sclera with a diathermy burn.*

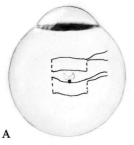

A

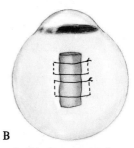

B

Figure 7–35. *Explant procedure. A. Diathermy mark on scleral surface identifies posterior border of retinal tear (shaded crescent); scleral mattress sutures are in place B Explant indented by the sutures.*

drainage of subretinal fluid. If this can be done, the scar will seal the retinal hole, and the subretinal fluid will absorb.

If there is a large amount of subretinal fluid, the eye may become very soft after fluid drainage. The implant will take up some of the space but, even after indentation of the implant, the eye often remains soft. Intravitreal injection is then indicated, to restore normal intraocular tension. Either fluid or gas may be injected (Fig. 7–38A). Any sterile balanced salt solution is satisfactory if a fluid is to be used. This solution will eventually be replaced by an aqueous-like fluid produced by the eye. Air is the most frequently used gas. A moderate sized air bubble (8 mm in diameter) will usually absorb within one week. It also will be re-

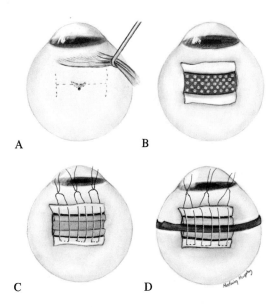

Figure 7–36. *Implant procedures. A. Diathermy mark(black dot) on surface of sclera identifies posterior border of retinal tear (shaded crescent.) Dotted lines indicate proposed partial-thickness scleral incision. B. Partial-thickness scleral flaps have been dissected. Diathermy applications are seen in the bed of the dissection. C. Mattress sutures have been inserted through the flaps. The implant lies in the bed. D. The encircling band has been placed through the groove in the implant. Everything is ready for drainage of subretinal fluid and closure of the sutures.*

placed by an aqueous-like fluid. Air can also be used to help reposition a retina that is not fully reattached at surgery (Fig. 7–38B). By positioning the patient so that the area of the retina needing to be moved toward the choroid is uppermost, gravity will allow the air to rise and press against the retina. Occasionally it will be desirable to maintain an intraocular gas bubble for longer than air will remain. Sulfahexofluride gas has been demonstrated to be nontoxic and is absorbed about twice as slowly as air.

Injections into the vitreous cavity are performed through the pars plana. The area on the surface of the globe that corresponds to the pars plana is a ring with its posterior edge at the muscle

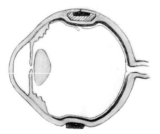

Figure 7–37. *Cross section of postscleral buckle eye. Note retina is flat and tear is on flat portion of implant. The encircling band is seen on the opposite side of the eye.*

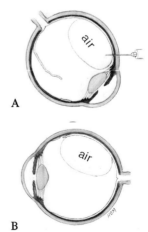

A

B

Figure 7–38. *Air injection. A. Use of air and gravity to flatten retinal tear. B. Head is positioned so that the air rises and presses retina against choroid.*

insertions and its width about 3.5 to 5 mm. A small-gauge needle, usually 30 gauge, is directed toward the center of the globe. Care must be taken not to strike the lens if the patient has one. If a larger needle is used, a mattress suture is placed across the injection site to close it after the needle is withdrawn.

RESULTS

About 20 percent of the time, the retina operation is unsuccessful in reattaching the retina. Usually, additional operations can be performed, but about 10 percent of retinal detachments are never cured.

The visual return following successful retinal detachment surgery depends on several things. If the macula is not involved in the detachment, it is likely that good vision will remain. The macula is the most sensitive area of the retina and the most susceptible to loss of choroidal nutrition. Once the macula has detached, it is impossible to predict the extent of visual return when the retina is reattached. However, it is well accepted that the longer the

macula is detached, and the higher that it is detached, the poorer
will be the visual return. Thus, retina operations are emergencies
if the macula is about to be involved in a detachment or if it has
just detached. The operation becomes less urgent the longer the
macula has been detached. The peripheral vision will return
unless the retina has been detached for many months. If, however,
the vision is reduced to no light perception preoperatively, the
retina has degenerated beyond recovery and operative intervention
is useless.

Preoperative Nursing Care

Patients who have been diagnosed as having a retinal detachment
are usually admitted the day that the retinal surgeon has made the
diagnosis. These patients are anxious and apprehensive. Generally
they have had some rapid loss of vision. Blindness or the fear of
losing sight is more of a reality to these people because of this sudden loss. You may hear the patient say, "This is a serious operation. My doctor tells me Dr. (retinal surgeon's name) is very
good, that he's the best there is. Dr. (retinal surgeon) says he does
many patients who have a similar problem to mine and usually
they need only one operation and that their vision is like it was
before they developed this eye problem." Some patients go
further to say, "I hope I don't have any difficulty," or "I don't
know what I'd do if I were blind." Others may stop short of
verbalizing this fear. We feel all patients need reassurance and
explanations in regard to their surgical procedure and its probable
outcome. Generally these patients have never met the retinal
surgeon previously because he is a consultant, and the confidence
and trust that they have with their general ophthalmologist is
transferred with some reservations to this "new doctor." Nurses
working with retinal patients can do much to allay apprehension
by reinforcing the possibility of a favorable outcome, and answering the patient's questions truthfully.

It has been our policy not to misrepresent the outcome; if it is
dubious, we indicate this to the patient. We try to instill hope, but
not false hope since we feel this makes a poor prognosis more
difficult for the patient to accept. Because the patient generally
has not had time to get ready for hospitalization, he may be very
anxious over general hospital procedures and routine. An orientation to the immediate environment is helpful. Taking time
to permit the patient to discuss the "eye problem," when the first,

symptoms developed, and how he came to being admitted can aid in relieving tension

In admitting a patient to the hospital and placing him on bedrest with bathroom privileges, one limits activities. This limited activity is helpful because the patient's vision is usually reduced. Thus he is less likely to fall and injure himself and perhaps cause more damage to the retina. This is particularly important if only part of the retina is detached; a fall or bump may cause a larger area of the retina to detach, and surgery would then be more difficult. Limitation of activity is even more important if the macula is not detached, since visual results are significantly better if the macula is not detached preoperatively. If the retina is totally detached, there is probably little need for limiting activity, unless the vision in the patient's other eye is poor.

The pupil is dilated with a mydriatic and a cycloplegic eyedrop. The mydriatic can be a drug such as phenylephrine hydrochloride (Neo-Synephrine 10%); the cycloplegic can be a drug such as cyclopentolate hydrochloride (Cyclogyl 1%), atropine 1%, scopolamine 0.25%, or homatropine. This dilatation achieves two purposes: (1) it permits the availability of examining the retina at any time; and (2) it prevents iritis, which is frequently associated with detachments, from binding the pupil in a constricted state and thereby prohibiting any future dilatation of that pupil.

Today most ophthalmologists have an internist evaluate the patient prior to surgery. Routine blood and urine studies are done. Patients over 40 years of age have an ECG taken. If a general anesthetic is planned, patients have a chest x-ray.

Bed rest with binocular eyepatches is utilized when it is felt that this maneuver would flatten the retina and lessen the manipulation at the time of surgery. Unilateral preoperative patching of the affected eye is not beneficial. Binocular patches are needed to prevent eye movements because the eyes move simultaneously. Patients are permitted bathroom privileges. The head of the bed may also be elevated for meals as long as the patches are in place.

Preoperative medications vary with the individual surgeon. Usually a narcotic, a sedative, and a narcotic potentiator or tranquilizer are given. An example of a frequently given preoperative medication would be meperidine (Demerol) 75 mg, and hydroxyzine pamoate (Vistaril) 50 mg given intramuscularly one hour preoperatively. Pentobarbital (Nembutal) 100 mg orally may be given 1½ hours preoperatively. Atropine is given intramuscularly to reduce secretions if the patient is to have a general anesthetic.

We do not use atropine intramuscularly preoperatively for local procedures because it dries the patient's nose and throat and makes him uncomfortable during surgery.

The mydriatic and cycloplegic eyedrops are instilled preoperatively as well as an antibiotic eyedrop to reduce the pathogens in the conjunctiva.

Postoperative Nursing Care

Postoperative nursing care is the same as for any surgical patient. Vital signs of blood pressure, pulse, and respiration should be taken every 15 minutes until stable then once every shift for 24 hours.

Patients return from the operating room with one or both eyes patched. The operated eye is always patched for cleanliness and patient comfort. Some surgeons prefer to patch both eyes following surgery. The theory is that if both eyes are patched they will move less, and, if any subretinal fluid should remain at the end of the operation, the retina will be more likely to settle against the choroid. The patch is removed from the unoperated eye when the retina settles against the choroid.

Most surgeons do not use binocular patches if the retina is flat at the end of the operation. However, some feel the retina will stay against the choroid more securely if the eyes are binocularly patched for two or three days. Safety precautions are essential if binocular patching is used. Assistance with all aspects of nursing care are indicated. An explanation of the immediate environment is indicated if binocular patching was not done preoperatively.

Postoperative dilatation of the pupil is maintained with a mydriatic and a cycloplegic. A combination of an eyedrop antibiotic and corticosteroid is given to reduce inflammation and to lower pathogens in the conjunctiva. These drops are instilled four times a day.

Edema and discomfort of the eyelids vary with individuals and with the amount of manipulation that was necessary in surgery to approximate the retina against the choroid. When removing the eyepatch to instill the eyedrops, you may see the eyes and eyelids so swollen that the conjunctiva is edematous and is peeking through the swollen lids. This may frighten the inexperienced nurse, who might feel that something has surely gone amiss, but this swelling will subside. You may also find, when removing the patch, that the eyes appear to be glued or sutured shut. These crusts and the serosanguineous discharge should be removed from the lashes with sterile saline or water. You may note a moderate to large amount of drainage for 24 to 48 hours post-operatively. Cold compresses are ordered at least four times a day to relieve this chemosis and ecchymosis as well as for lid comfort and cleanliness. Having the eye patched and at rest also assists in reducing this edema.

Deep breathing is instituted 15 times every hour if the patient has had a general anesthetic. For all patients, passive and active range of motion exercises are utilized to prevent formation of thrombi.

Activity orders for patients vary. Most patients are permitted bathroom privileges the day of surgery and thereafter. They may have a pillow. Elevation of the head of the bed for meals may vary from 30° to 90°. On the third postoperative day the patient may be up and walking.

Pain or discomfort in the operated eye varies. Frequently, patients describe this as a temporal or frontal headache. Medications vary depending on severity of discomfort. Meperidine (Demerol) 50 to 100 mg, acetaminophen with codeine (Tylenol) one or two No. 3 tablets, or Tylenol, one or two gr X tablets is administered as needed to give relief.

Postoperative nausea and vomiting varies with individual patients. An antiemetic is ordered and generally suffices to relieve the discomfort.

Air or balanced salt solution can be injected into the vitreous cavity to inflate a collapsed globe. The patient is positioned so that the air will mechanically press against the area where the chorioretinitis has been made. Since air rises, the patient is positioned so that the area of the retina that needs to be flattened is uppermost. The surgeon indicates the exact position of head placement. If the area to be affected by the air is at the posterior pole, the patient may lie flat (prone position) with the head face down and turned slightly on a small pillow or a folded bath blanket (Fig. 7–39). Since the patient may remain in this position for four or five days, until the air is absorbed, the position becomes tedious and tiring for the patient. As the nurse, you want to remember that the patient can be in any position as long as his head remains parallel to the floor and the air is at the posterior pole. Therefore, the patient can sit in a Fowler's position, with his head resting on an overbed table which can be adjusted for the patient's height (Fig. 7–40). Aphakic patients who have air injected

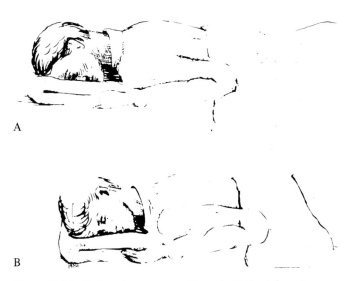

Figure 7–39. *Patient in prone position. A. Patient face down to position air bubble at posterior pole. B. Patient face turned slightly to position air bubble temporal to the posterior pole.*

into the vitreous cavity should not lie on their backs for long periods of time. This would cause the air to rise, pushing the iris forward, and closing off the angle, thus causing an acute glaucoma. Patients with lenses should not lie on their backs for long periods of time because air in contact with the lens may cause a cataract.

Discharge teaching should begin on the first postoperative day or at the earliest possible time. Discharge usually is five to seven days after surgery. Physicians generally request patients to come for a postoperative visit one week after discharge. Patients are discharged with two eyedrops, a cycloplegic, and an anti-inflammatory, antibiotic type drop to be instilled four times a day.

Patients should avoid being in crowds or in unfamiliar places so as to avoid falling or undue jostling. Reading, which involves rapid, jerky eye movements as the eye travels from the end of one line to the next should be limited. Watching television, which does not involve so many jerky eye movements, is permissible, since watching television is straight-ahead vision. Patients may do light housework such as some light dusting, but should not move or lift heavy furniture, vacuum, or scrub. In two weeks the patient may return to sedentary work. In six weeks, heavy work and

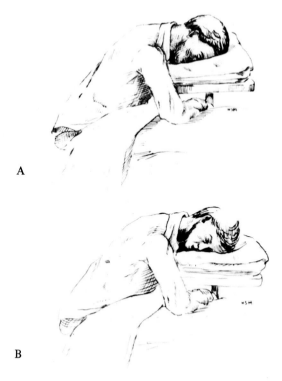

A

B

Figure 7–40. *Patient in Fowler's position. A. Patient face down to position air bubble at posterior pole. B. Patient face turned slightly to position air bubble temporal to the posterior pole of right eye.*

athletic activities, such as tennis or contact sports, can be permitted. Tennis should be avoided before six weeks because of the danger of being hit with the ball. Refractions are done in approximately three months.

Patients who have noticed preoperative floaters may complain of these postoperatively, since reattaching the retina does not remove the vitreous opacities. Also those who did not notice floaters preoperatively because of poor vision may notice floaters when the retina is reattached and their vision improves. Usually floaters absorb rapidly but they may persist for years until the blood is reabsorbed or the floaters drop inferiorly below the visual axis.

The continuation of light flashes indicates that all vitreous traction was not relieved by surgery. This does not mean that the retinal surgery was not successful, or that detachment will recur, but it probably indicates continued vitreous disturbance and is a warning to the surgeon to watch this eye closely in the post-operative period.

Floaters and light flashes may not be noticed until the patient goes home, at which point they become alarmed and call the retinal surgeon's office, receiving some alleviation of their anxiety from the nurse clinician. Others will notice this during hospitalization and receive support from the nurse giving tertiary care.

RETROLENTAL FIBROPLASIA

Retrolental fibroplasia is a disease of premature infants and causes retinal detachment in its more advanced stages. The disease rarely occurs unless oxygen is administered to the premature infant.

The disease occurs in premature infants because the retinal vasculature has not completely developed. Vascularization of the retina begins in the early fetal life at the optic disc and progresses peripherally at an equal rate until the retina is entirely vascularized at full term. If premature birth occurs, the normal progression usually occurs after birth unless oxygen must be given to save the infant's life. High arterial oxygen tension, > 60 mm Hg, will cause contraction of the small peripheral arterial tree. When normal oxygen tension returns, these vessels respond by overgrowth of vascular and fibrous tissue resulting in traction on the retina. These changes more commonly occur on the temporal side of the eye, since complete vascularization occurs about one to two months later than on the nasal side. The result varies from minimal preretinal fibrosis in the temporal periphery to total inoperable traction retinal detachment and fibrosis. A very common finding is the presence of a retinal fold extending from the disc through the macula and to the temporal periphery. This has been termed *dragged disc* and is pathognomonic of this condition (see Fig. 7-41).

Prevention is the best treatment. This requires repeated arterial oxygen calculations on any premature infant under oxygen therapy. There is no satisfactory clinical method of evaluating arterial oxygen tension. Skin color indicates whether the infant is getting too little oxygen but not whether he is getting too much. Blood absorption is dependent on the maturity of the lung

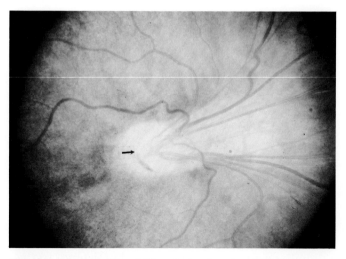

Figure 7–41. *Retrolental fibroplasia, showing vessels dragged temporally. Macula is hidden in the grayish retinal folds. Arrow points to nasal side of disc. (Photo courtesy of Frank Flanagin, Associated Retinal Consultants, Detroit.)*

tissue, and, thus, oxygen concentration of the inspired air is unreliable.

Surgical repair of localized peripheral detachments is effective. However, the massive total detachments have been generally untreatable. Although children with the dragged disc will have side vision, no treatment is available to improve the central (reading) vision.

RETINOSCHISIS

Retinoschisis means splitting of the retina. The initial appearance is that of a retinal detachment. However, schisis is like a cyst of the retina since the retina is split just inside the rod-and-cone layer. Retinoschisis is more prevalent in the elderly, invariably begins in the periphery, and usually does not progress beyond the equator. It may develop retinal holes and lead to a retinal detachment. Therefore, treatment is indicated when holes develop. Usually, cryothermy alone is sufficient treatment. The cyst collapses and the holes are sealed.

CHOROIDAL DETACHMENT

Fluid can develop between the choroid and the sclera. This is
called a *choroidal detachment.* Choroidal detachments usually
occur following intraocular surgery or long-standing intraocular
inflammatory disease. This is particularly common if the eye
becomes soft. The fluid can be a transudate from choroidal vessels or blood.

In most cases spontaneous reabsorption occurs. Systemic or
subconjunctival steroids have been recommended, but their effect
is unpredictable. Surgical drainage can be performed by making
an incision through the sclera about 5 to 10 mm behind the
corneal limbus. Saline or air must then be injected into the vitreous
cavity to normalize intraocular pressure.

APPENDIX I
Modifications On Insulin Techniques
For The Visually Impaired Or Blind Diabetic*

by
Alice Raftary, B.S., M.Ed.
Supervisor of Teaching and
Personal Adjustment Training
GREATER DETROIT SOCIETY FOR THE BLIND
December, 1976

CAUTION!
This is not a complete insulin instruction. It is concerned with technique modification and presumes a considerable knowledge of diabetes and insulin management. Persons with a non-medical background should use this booklet with the consultation of an experienced nurse or clinician. Improper interpretation of insulin prescription can have serious consequences. It should be noted that insulin is a potentially lethal drug.

MAKING THE TEMPLET

A templet provides a simple, easily handled, accurate measuring device for the insulin dose. One may be simply and economically made of refill staples and a soft adhesive tape (masking, Mystic, surgical, etc.).
Directions: Set the dose on the syringe. Break off a length of staples slightly longer than the length of exposed plunger. Remove a few staples at a time, until the length of staples fits snugly between the exposed plunger end and the syringe barrel. Wrap the length of staples, including one of the angles, with tape to insure permanence and rigidity. Check the accuracy of the templet.
Note: A new templet must be made if there is any change in prescription or in the make or model of syringe.

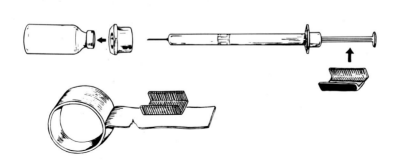

INSERTING THE NEEDLE INTO THE INSULIN VIAL

In the dominant hand, hold the syringe near the needle hub as a pencil. With the other hand, hold the insulin vial firmly upright on the table, thumb and forefinger at the neck of the vial.

As the needle is brought to rest across the vial top, the free fingers of the hand holding the syringe will help locate the vial and steady the hand.

Draw the needle across the vial cap. There will be a small click as the tip comes off the metal ring onto the rubber. Rotate the syringe to the perpendicular and insert it into the vial. If the needle is not on the rubber, there will be resistance. Don't force it, as the needle will bend. Start over.

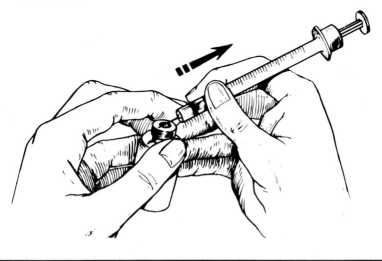

TECHNIQUE FOR DRAWING UP INSULIN

Assemble all equipment on a small, shallow tray or box.

Mix insulin by rolling the vial gently between the palms of the hands.

Cleanse the vial cap with an alcohol swab. Return swab to tray.

Uncover the needle. After the needle is uncovered, the syringe does not leave the hands until it is ready for disposal. Draw air into the syringe to the amount of the insulin dose by placing the templet along the shaft of the plunger and seating it snugly. Remove the templet and return it to the tray for easy relocation.

With the vial resting firmly upright on the table, insert the needle. Expel the air into the vial.

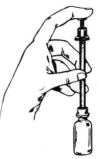

Slowly invert the vial with syringe attached. Hold it in a vertical position in one hand, leaving the dominant hand free to manipulate the plunger. Keep the equipment in a vertical position until the insulin is fully drawn.

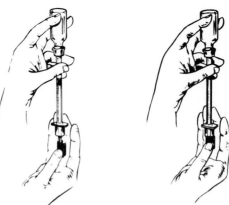

With the dominant hand, pull out the plunger approximately ¼″ farther than necessary to insert the templet. Position the templet along the plunger shaft. Push the plunger up so that the templet is seated. The insulin in the syringe is the dosage prescribed.

ADDITIONAL PROCEDURES FOR TWO INSULINS IN A SINGLE DOSE

Make two templets. One templet should be made to measure the units drawn first. The other templet is the length of the combined dose. Be sure the insulins can be differentiated tactually (e.g., a rubber band around one of the vials).

Draw up air with the longer templet to the combined dose.

Remove templet and insert needle in vial of insulin to be drawn second.

Place the small templet along the shaft of the plunger, and expel air into the vial until the small templet is seated.

Withdraw syringe with templet still in place.

Insert needle into the vial of insulin to be drawn first.

Draw up the first part of the dose, following the procedures described in this manual.

Remove the needle from the vial, keeping the templet in place. Return the vial to the tray.

Keeping the templet in place, insert the needle into the second vial.

Invert the vial, and remove the small templet, drawing up a few units.

Set the longer templet with the end resting on the end of the plunger, and carefully pull out the plunger, steadying the templet with the thumb until the templet drops into place and is seated. Do not expel any insulin back into the second vial.

Withdraw the syringe from the vial with templet in place. If extra insulin was drawn, discard it by seating the templet.

Remove the templet and proceed with injection.

TECHNIQUE FOR INJECTION

With the free hand, pick up the alcohol swab between the fingers, leaving the thumb and index finger free. Use the swab to cleanse the injection site.

Keeping the swab between the fingers, pinch up the cleansed area between the index finger and the thumb.

Place the needle at the injection site. The needle should be at a slight angle, lightly touching the skin. Do not jab. The syringe is then pivoted so that it is nearly perpendicular to the flesh.

Insert the needle and inject the insulin.

Bring the alcohol swab to the needle. As the needle is withdrawn, press the site with alcohol swab.

Cover the needle and dispose of the syringe.

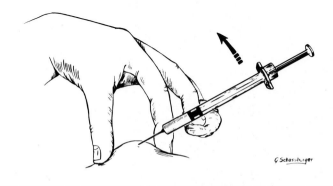

*From Alice Raftary, Greater Detroit Society for the Blind. Used with permission.

SELECTED READINGS

BOOKS

Duke-Elder, S., (Ed.). *System of Ophthalmology,* Vol. 10. Diseases of the Retina. St. Louis: Mosby, 1967.

Guthrie, D. W., and Richard, A. (Eds.). *Nursing Management of Diabetes Mellitus.* St. Louis: Mosby, 1977.

Kimura, S. J., and Caygell, W. M. (Eds.). *Retinal Disease.* Philadelphia: Lea & Febiger, 1966.

ARTICLES

Porter, A. L. (Guest Ed.). Symposium on diabetes patient education and care. *Nursing Clinics of North America* 12(3): 407–414, 1977.

Smith, J. F., and Nachazel, D. P. Retinal detachment. *American Journal of Nursing.* 73(9): 1530–1535, 1973.

PART II

CARE OF THE VISUALLY HANDICAPPED

CHAPTER 8

NURSING CARE AND REHABILITATION OF THE VISUALLY HANDICAPPED

The visual disability, blindness, is a sensory loss dreaded by most individuals. The inability to see our immediate surroundings, the size of the room, the color of the chair or walls, the characteristics of the person to whom one is speaking makes us uneasy. We need only to close our eyes and grope around our own living room to realize how difficult and frightening this experience can be.

There are two categories of patients with visual disabilities: those who have been born blind and those who have lost sight through disease or accident. In this chapter we will refer to the latter category, those who have had sight and lost it through disease or accident. This section will stress some helpful hints and measures for the nurse or family to institute before a rehabilitation program is begun for the newly disabled. Also we have tried to stress some nursing measures to assist in making hospitalization a positive experience.

ORIENTATION

The person who has lost sight will have a background knowledge of concepts that can be utilized to assist him in becoming oriented to his environment. For instance, you can describe the room by giving its size. If the patient cannot judge size, you could walk him the length and the width of the room. In describing a room, it is best to pick a focal point. The patient's bed should be the focal point of the hospital room. You must describe the position of the bed in relation to the other major items within the room. Begin as you enter the room, describing how to reach the bed from the door. Then walk into the room and stand at the foot of the bed with the patient so that he can place his hands on the footboard. This will make the bed the focal point of the room. Patients should never be left in the middle of a room, but near a piece of furniture or next to a wall. You can then describe the room in this fashion, "Now we are standing at the foot of the bed, and on the

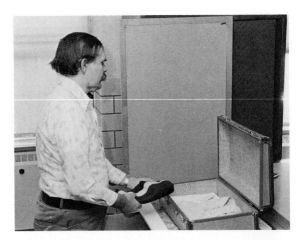

Figure 8-1. *Patients should be permitted to unpack clothes themselves when admitted to the hospital. (Photo courtesy of Frank Flanagin, Associated Retinal Consultants, Detroit.)*

left-hand side of the bed, as you face it, is an armchair. On the right-hand side of the bed is your nightstand. Standing next to the nightstand is a straight back chair. Two feet from the chair on the right wall is your closet. Next to that on the closet's right is your bathroom." While doing this, walk with the patient to the object being described so that the patient can use his hands to aid in examining his environment.

In assisting the patient to unpack you could direct him to stand in front of the nightstand, permitting him to run his hand over its circumference to judge its size. It is advisable to let the patient place his belongings in the drawer (Fig. 8-1). This enables him to function more satisfactorily, as he is aware of placement and can help himself to whatever personal articles are needed. After the patient and you unpack his belongings, you may describe the bathroom. Include in your discussion the placement of the toilet, toilet tissue dispenser, washbowl, and bathtub.

It is important that the individual patient's care plan include the placement of phone, water pitcher, call light, and television or radio controls. These items should remain in a constant position. It is nice if the patient does not have to remind the personnel of placement of needed equipment dozens of times during the hospital stay.

If the patient chooses to use the telephone frequently, learning to dial by himself may bring a feeling of independence that will

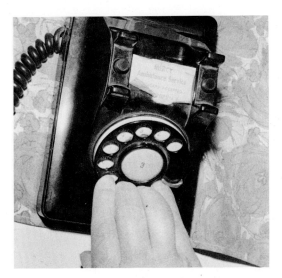

Figure 8-2. *One position for dialing: little finger 0, ring finger 9, middle finger 8, index finger 7 (phone is a right-handed instrument). (Photo courtesy of Frank Flanagin, Associated Retinal Consultants, Detroit.)*

"lift his spirits." The general procedure for dialing the phone is for the patient to place the little finger of his right hand in the number 1, the ring finger in 2, the middle finger in 3, and the index finger in 4. By reaching the index finger downward, the patient finds 5. He then removes his hand and moves the little finger to 0, the ring finger to 9, the middle finger to 8, and the index finger to 7. By reaching the index finger up one space, he finds 6. This hand placement is in general use by all rehabilitation centers (Fig. 8–2). It is similar to learning a standard hand placement for a typewriter. Hence, the general method of dialing would be reinforced by the rehabilitation team if the patient were to remain permanently disabled or be blind from his eye disease.

If the patient is unable to dial for himself or becomes too "upset" at trying to dial, the Bell telephone company has an "0 service" (operator service) for blind patients. The advent of Centrex systems in medical centers makes getting a hospital operator difficult. Patients become frustrated over their repeated failures to dial out or to get assistance from the hospital-based operator. When such problems occur, the nursing staff should notify the

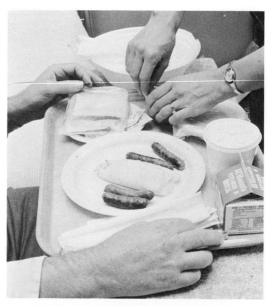

Figure 8-3. *Nurse assists the patient in setting up his breakfast tray. (Photo courtesy of Frank Flanagin, Associated Retinal Consultants, Detroit.)*

hospital operator who in turn notifies the telephone company that a blind patient is in the hospital and will need 0 service. Once the operator has the patient's phone number, the 0 service can commence. This protocol may not be identical in all institutions, and therefore, you should check to see what service is available for the handicapped. When patients are discharged, they may do the same thing with their residential phone by simply dialing 0 and indicating that they need 0 service. This type of service to the blind is available throughout the United States.

Patients usually enjoy being able to eat without assistance. The clock placement of food can be utilized. It is best for the nurse to cut food, butter bread, or pour coffee (Fig. 8-3). With modern disposable containers the nurse may open the juice container only halfway so that the patient will not spill the contents. In due time, patients who are going to be permanently blind must learn this skill, but it is difficult and frustrating at first. The patient may have just learned of his loss of sight and not be able to immediately "muster the desire" to be rehabilitated. The mourning or

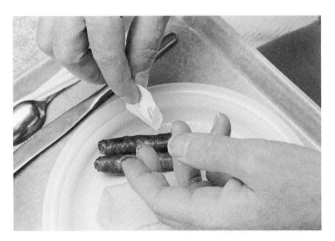

Figure 8-4. *Condiments are smelled to differentiate salt from pepper. Note: They are then run through the fingers to estimate the amount placed on food. (Photo courtesy of Frank Flanagin, Associated Retinal Consultants, Detroit.)*

grief period can be interlocked with hostility, anger, helplessness, and fear. If the patient is pushed into trying to pour, cut food, and judge amounts of food on a knife or spoon (such as amount of sugar or jelly on a spoon, or of butter on the spreader) he may become frustrated, begin crying, and not be able to eat. Patients are taught to smell condiments such as salt, pepper, catsup, or mustard. Salt or pepper is shaken over the fingertips for the person to estimate the amount being placed on his food (Fig. 8–4).

In some instances, patients may be permitted to eat in a dining room. If the patient is taken to the dining room, he should be left standing behind his chair. He will then run his hands over the surface of the top of the back of the chair and also over the seat of the chair. Holding the back of the chair, he will move his hand from the chair to the table to judge the distance. After seating himself (always permit the patient to pull out his own chair and seat himself), he will take his hands and trail the table identifying his plate and silverware. In trailing, the patient uses the dorsal (back) side of the index and middle fingers, running them along the surface he is examining. He will trail in a slow, deliberate, but inconspicuous way to avoid spilling. He will, if experienced, identify his food by using his fork and knife. Generally, patients

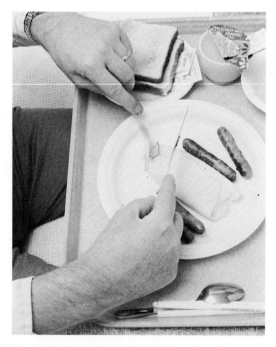

Figure 8-5. *Food is felt with the side of the fork, and utensils are held European style. Note orange juice container is half open to avoid spilling. (Most commercial companies fill glasses to the brim.) (Photo courtesy of Frank Flanagin, Associated Retinal Consultants, Detroit.)*

are taught to use the European method with the fork in the left hand and the knife in the right—as it is more acceptable than using one's hand as a pusher for food (Fig. 8-5).

MOBILITY TRAINING

WITH A GUIDE

In assisting a visually disabled patient to walk, permit him to take your arm. Do not take his arm and begin pulling him down the hall. The patient will utilize the three-point hold to grasp your arm at the elbow, with his thumb, index finger, and middle finger to hold your arm (Fig. 8-6). As the guide, you should keep your arm close to your body, for the patient to feel the direction that

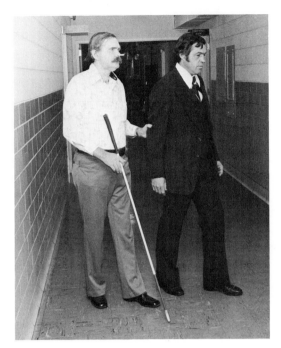

Figure 8–6. *Method for leading the blind. Note: Leader's arm is held close to his side, the blind person grasps just above the elbow. (Photo courtesy of Frank Flanagin, Associated Retinal Consultants, Detroit.)*

your body is moving. Frequently, the patient will keep one step behind the guide or mobility instructor. The patient is told that when approaching a narrow doorway or a crowded area, the guide will drop his arm behind him, in that way alerting the patient to walk behind the guide. When the guide moves his arm back to his side the patient can again move to the guide's side.

The guide or nurse should be sure to give the patient warning of obstacles in his path. Nurses should be aware of the need for in-service education and continued reassessment of the nursing staff's ability to aid in mobility of the visually handicapped. Nurses need to warn patients of narrow passageways, furniture that is protruding in their path, or forthcoming steps. Particular patient problems can be indicated for each individual on the Kardex, such as hesitancy to go down steps or other problems encountered while in the hospital.

WITH A CANE

Many blind patients are now receiving mobility training. This involves instruction in the use of a long white stick, called the *long white cane.* This cane is not used for support. It is used to feel the terrain in front of the patient and thus permit him to walk in unfamiliar territory without assistance. The cane, when held vertically, should reach the base of the sternum, give or take an inch. Thus the cane is about chest height in length. The cane is always held in the center of the body and is never raised more than two inches from the floor. For walking, the tip of the cane should strike the floor on the right side outside of the shoulder as the left foot is touching the floor (Fig. 8–7). The cane then moves in a swinging arc about two inches from the floor to touch the floor on the outside of the left shoulder as the right foot is touching the floor. In this way, the cane is always examining the area where the patient's foot will next fall or preparing the way for the next footstep. The patient must learn to stop quickly without losing his balance when the cane strikes an object. Inability to stop quickly could cause the patient to injure himself by falling or by bumping into objects. If the patient is hospitalized, the nurse should assist him in obtaining points of reference. These points of reference will assist him in orienting himself to his immediate environment. These may be doorways, depressions in the wall, or areas jutting out of the wall. Stairways or elevators should be included in your clues to the patient.

TRAILING

Patients frequently use trailing to orient themselves for moving about as well as for eating. For instance, if the patient is standing in the middle of a room, guide him to a wall or a chair. He can then trail by using the dorsal side of the index and middle fingers and run them along the wall. In doing this the patient should hold his opposite arm in flexion position at the face level (Fig. 8–8). With this technique the patient can explore his own room without injuring himself. When the patient begins mobility training he is taught to trail with one hand and to run the cane along the baseboard in front of him for protection. Figure 8–9 illustrates this situation.

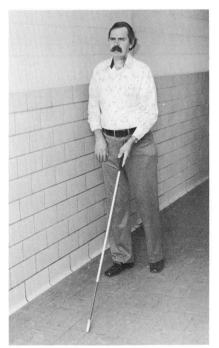
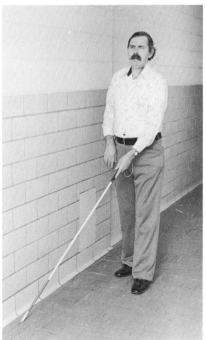

A   B

Figure 8-7. *Mobility with cane. A. Cane clearing way for left foot. B. Cane clearing way for right foot. (Photo courtesy of Frank Flanagin, Associated Retinal Consultants, Detroit.)*

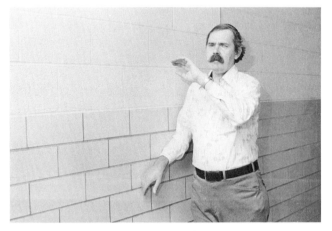

Figure 8-8. *Examining the room. Left arm protects face, right arm trails wall. (Photo courtesy of Frank Flanagin, Associated Retinal Consultants, Detroit.)*

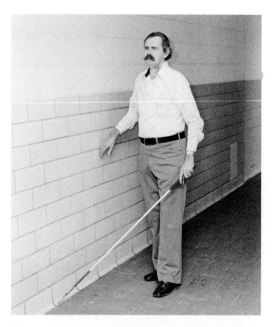

Figure 8–9. *Beginning mobility with cane. Hand is used to trail wall. Long white cane is used to run along the side of floorboard and slightly in front of patient for protection. (Photo courtesy of Frank Flanagin, Associated Retinal Consultants, Detroit.)*

LOW-VISION AIDS

Low-vision clinics help to assist patients to utilize any existing vision. The severely visually disabled patient has numerous types of symptoms including distortion, blurring, and haziness. The aim of low-vision equipment would be to magnify as well as to make clear a portion or segment of material. In this way, the patient could scan and possibly visualize a total object or read a total paragraph. The aim or goal of any low-vision aid is to provide visual compensation that will suffice to assist the patient in performing as many activities requiring vision as possible. The optical device can be in the form of spectacles, hand lenses, or telescopic lenses. There can be any number of a variety of aids utilized; for example, spectacles and prisms can be used for some patients whose vision is not too low.

I still find each day too short for all the thoughts I want to think, all the walks I want to take, all the books I want to read, and all the friends I want to see. The longer I live the more my mind dwells upon the beauty and the wonder of the world.

John Burroughs

A

I still find each day too short for all the thoughts I want to think, all the walks I want to take, all the books I want to read, and all the friends I want to see. The longer I live the more my mind dwells upon the beauty and the wonder of the world.

John Burroughs

B

Figure 8–10. *A. Standard type size. B. Large type size for the visually handicapped.*

There are numerous aids to improve the quality of life of patients with low vision. Popular books and educational texts have been transcribed to phonograph records and tape decks. Volunteers for associations for the blind record books for individual patient's needs, be they personal or educational.

Some materials are printed in large type (e.g., the *Reader's Digest* and *The New York Times,* as well as some versions of the bible). Figure 8–10 shows the difference between the two sizes of print.

Some helpful aids can assist patients in being more independent and capable of transacting their own business, for example, a

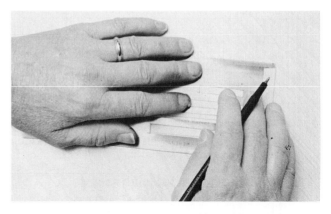

Figure 8-11. *Template for check writing. (Photo courtesy of Frank Flanagin, Associated Retinal Consultants, Detroit.)*

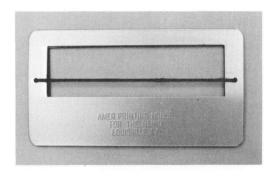

Figure 8-12. *A signature template, which a blind person can easily carry in his pocket. (Photo courtesy of Frank Flanagin, Associated Retinal Consultants, Detroit.)*

template for writing, which can easily be made to adapt to an individual's checkbook or to writing paper (Figs. 8-11, 8-12, 8-13). These are only a few examples of aids to assist patients in enjoying an independent life.

It has been said that the patient must "die as a sighted person in order to be reborn as a blind man." He must accept the fact that he is now a different person, and that he will have a new or different way of living. Patients must and can learn all activities of daily living. This takes time, patience, determination, and courage.

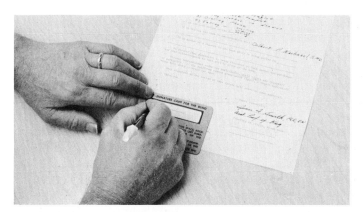

Figure 8-13. *Signature template in place for patient to sign. (Photo courtesy of Frank Flanagin, Associated Retinal Consultants, Detroit.)*

REHABILITATION CENTERS

Many valuable hints and much assistance can be obtained through the rehabilitation center. Blind patients are assisted to work through problems to realize that indeed life is worth living, but that it is a different life. Each patient is an individual with different potentials and different levels of achievement, each striving to become an independent, productive member of society.

Rehabilitation centers conduct programs that last three months or longer to assist patients to learn a new way of living down to the small details of daily life. They are equipped to pass on many helpful hints—for example, how to mark clothing so that colors are coordinated and socks are in pairs. (A simple method is different embroidery stitches or patterns of knots inside collars or on the inside of the waistbands.) The center will assist in determining ways to fold paper money so that bills can be easily sorted and identified.

BLIND PATIENTS

When patients are bilaterally eyepatched or blind, we ask our staff to knock on the door before entering the patient's room. This not only gives the patient warning that someone is entering, to avoid frightening him, but also imparts the feeling that this is his space. The immediate surroundings then have a personal touch, giving each patient a feeling of his bed and his area of the unit.

When entering we give our name immediately and tell the patient what we will be doing for him that day. It is devastating for the patient to be trying to guess with whom he is conversing. Each time one enters he should repeat his name.

We visit the patient five minutes out of every hour if possible, to have a short conversation, or to check on how the patient is feeling. Patients are encouraged to listen to the news, their favorite talk shows, or music. We feel that asking the patient to use his memory by telling us what was on the news at 7 A.M. assists him in remaining oriented. If a patient regularly listens to a specific program, his listening assists in orienting him to time. Because the patients may easily doze off, we remind them of the time and day each shift. This helps them to keep the days in order. However, if a patient sleeps frequently and does not listen to the radio or to a talk show, he frequently becomes confused with the time of day or whether it is the same day or the following day. A way to assist patients to be oriented to time is to buy an inexpensive clock and remove the glass face (Fig. 8–14). (The less expensive the clock, the easier to remove the face.) The patient can then feel the hands and note the time of day. Some patients need a piece of tape placed at the 12, 3, 6, and 9 position, and others have no difficulty.

When possible, we try to get the patient to plan his own care for the day. This assists in having him use his memory as well as to plan for the future occurrences during the day. When feasible. we discuss discharge planning and how the patient will care for himself at home.

The patient who has been temporarily blind is relieved when once again he joins the world of "the sighted." Many of these patients relieve their tensions by expressing their fears of blindness and their relief at being able to see, and to do for themselves again.

PARTIALLY SIGHTED PATIENTS

The visual disability of monocular vision or of the loss of vision in one eye can be quite disabling until the patient learns to adjust. The problems the patient must learn to overcome are loss of a full visual field and loss of depth perception. While these problems can be overcome, they can be quite annoying to the patient. These visual disturbances are the same whether they occur in a

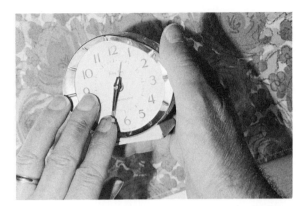

Figure 8-14. *Telling time. Clock face without glass.*
(Photo courtesy of Frank Flanagin, Associated Retinal
Consultants, Detroit.)

unilateral eyepatched patient, a patient blind in one eye, or a
patient with some visual loss in one eye.

With decreased or unilateral vision, one no longer has a visual
field of 180°+. The patient loses approximately 50° of peripheral
vision on the affected side. The loss is less than one-half of the
total visual field and occurs because the nasal field of each eye
overlaps. This loss of a full visual field requires adjustment on the
part of the patient. In social situations, he must pick a seat, where
he can conveniently turn and see all persons with whom he is
conversing. When crossing the street, he must turn his head and be
more careful, to protect himself from injury. When eating, he must
turn his head as he can miss a side dish of food or a beverage
placed on the affected side.

The loss of depth perception causes difficulty in judging dis-
tances or size of objects and is an annoyance. The person finds it
difficult to pour juice from a pitcher into a glass because he misjudges the position of the two objects. At times he misjudges the
distance of a chair and more or less "falls into" furniture that is at
a lower height than he anticipated. He has difficulty with steps,
judging the height of each one, as well as realizing that the last
step has been reached. The steps seemingly blend in with the
carpet. In older patients, the height of the curb often is misjudged
and the person lunges forward, falling or turning his ankle.

These problems are annoying to the patient, and an alert clinician can give some helpful guidelines to the patient depending
on the degree of his visual disability.

PATIENTS WITH LOW VISION

Patients who have poor vision need assistance with reorganizing their household. There are many helpful hints for homemakers. An area of difficulty is the kitchen. Refrigerators frequently have poor lighting. Often there is only one bulb, which does not illuminate all areas sufficiently for the person with decreased vision. Food that is in the back of the refrigerator can spoil or be overlooked. Labels are frequently missed, or the print is too small for the patient to read. Added lighting can be installed to shine on the labels and food containers. This may require a larger watt kitchen bulb or a portable extension light with a long cord, which can be utilized in various areas of the kitchen.

Kitchen cupboards also can be dark. Therefore finding staples and condiments can be a problem. Additional lighting is helpful.

If a patient is blind or has very low visual function, foods can be marked or identified by marking with tape, rubber bands, or by using various shaped containers for easy identification.

When patients have poor vision, it is difficult for them to see an object if the light, be it artificial or natural, is behind the object or person they are conversing with or looking toward. The object or person then is a shadow or has no specific characteristics. One should remember to have the light in front of the object or person he is viewing. Nurses working with the visually handicapped should remember this and place themselves conveniently. Patients who have a disability should be urged to situate themselves in a comfortable position and urged to change their seat if need be when in a group, to facilitate comfort in social conversation and social settings.

Patients with decreased vision have difficulty in viewing an identical color upon itself (white on white or green on green)—for instance, white bread crumbs on a white tablecloth or a green phone on a green formica countertop might be difficult to see. A hazardous situation would be the same color stair carpeting as the carpeting at the foot of the stairs. Additional lighting and hand rails can be of some help to the visually disabled. Redecorating by making color changes is helpful, if feasible. The sharper the contrast of color utilized, the easier it will be for the visually handicapped patient.

In this chapter we have tried to give some practical helpful assistance to help you assist patients with their visual disability. There is much need for assistance to be given to the patient with limited sight. Your awareness of the kinds of problems that can occur will assist you to look for new sources that will enrich the quality of your patient's life.

SELECTED READINGS

BOOKS

Brady, F. B. *A Singular View—The Art of Seeing Without One Eye.* Oradell, NJ: Medical Economics Co., 1972.

Faye, E. E., and Hood, C. M. *Low Vision.* Springfield, IL: Thomas, 1975.

Ross Round Table on Natural and Child Nursing. *Patients with Sensory Disturbances—Implications for Nursing Practice and Research.* Columbus, OH: Ross Laboratories, 1966.

ARTICLES

Downs, F. D. Bedrest and sensory disturbances. *American Journal of Nursing* 74: 434–437, 1974.

Jackson, W., and Ellis, R. Sensory deprivation. *Nursing Research* 20: 46–53, 1971.

Ohno, M. I. The eye-patched patient. *American Journal of Nursing* 71: 271–274, 1971.

Thompson, L. Sensory deprivation—A personal experience. *American Journal of Nursing* 73: 266–268, 1973.

We appreciate the help of Victor Irving, The Blind Services of the Rehabilitation Institute of Detroit, and of Cam Williams, Occupational Therapy of Detroit, for their suggestions and assistance in critically reading this chapter.

CHAPTER 9 ⸺

PHYSICAL ASSESSMENT

With the advent of new nursing roles such as primary care, extended practice, and nurse practitioners, the need for nurses to do physical assessments has increased. This new and important role can be helpful to the physician as well as the patient.

OBSERVATION OF PHYSICAL CHARACTERISTICS

Before beginning a physical assessment, a thorough history should be taken. Begin your physical assessment by observation.

POSTURE

Note the patient's appearance, his posture, head tilt, or any other noticeable postural characteristics that could be clues to compensatory stances to attain clear vision. For example, the patient who has double vision, such as with strabismus, may cock his head to the side to focus and to see a single object.

SYMMETRY

It is helpful to observe symmetry, such as the appearance of the left eye vs. the right eye. Observe the patient's facial symmetry. Note placement of the eyes. Are they placed an equal distance from one another? Observe the eyebrows. Is the growth of hair evenly distributed in both brows, or is there an absence of eyebrows? Any abnormality in the eyebrow is generally due to a dermatologic condition rather than an ophthalmic one. Can the patient raise or elevate the eyebrows? Inability to raise the eyebrows would indicate damage to the seventh cranial (facial) nerve.

EYELIDS AND CONJUNCTIVA

Observe the eyelid. Is there drooping or ptosis of the lid? Is there redness, tenderness, or swelling of the lid and lashes, such as a chalazion or a stye respectively. If a chalazion is thought to be present, the upper lid must be everted to examine the meibomian gland area and more readily confirm the diagnosis. You can see the meibomian glands as they exit on the margins of the eyelids. The meibomian glands are tubular and extend into the tarsal plate. The lower lid must be examined also, as the meibomian glands line both upper and lower lids. Pull down on the lower lid to examine the area.

To evert the upper eyelid, have the patient look down, asking him not to squeeze his eyelid (squeezing the eye contracts the orbicularis muscle and prevents you from everting the lid). Grasp the eyelashes, gently pulling downward. Place a cotton tip applicator on the skin side of the upper lid (See Fig. 10–1). While pushing down on the skin side of the lid (or pushing down on the upper tarsal border, flip the eyelid up over the applicator). Gentle pressure on upper lashes against the superior part of the lid will maintain eversion if the patient continues to look down (See Fig. 10–2).

While the upper lid is everted and the patient looks down (otherwise the lid will revert to its normal position), observe the superior temporal area of the palpebral fissure. If the lacrimal gland is enlarged, it will be seen in this area. Are there signs of inflammation, swelling, or redness? While the upper lid is everted, note the pale, glistening, pink conjunctiva. A very pale whitish conjunctiva can be a sign of a blood dyscrasia and may require further investigation. There is a wide range of normalcy, so blood counts should not be taken indiscriminately.

Check the punctum, which is in the nasal third of the lid margin. Observe for any swelling, redness or tenderness. Check the preauricular gland (usually this gland cannot be palpated) located superior to the condyle of the mandible. These structures can become involved if there is an infection of the lids or conjunctiva.

SCLERA

Observe the sclera. Is it white? If the sclera is turning yellow, this may be an indication of jaundice and systemic problems. A blue tinge usually indicates a thinned sclera, and is a result of the choroid showing through the sclera. Bluish sclera is common in the newborn because of the normally thin sclera, but otherwise is rare. Infections of the sclera can occur but are rare.

CORNEA

Check the cornea. Is it clear? The cornea is the transparent area covering the iris, or colored part of the eye. At times, some cloudy area or specks can be observed on the cornea; these can be from accidents or injuries. Cataracts in the early stages also appear as small cloudy areas, but they are seen behind the pupil.

MUSCLES

Next have the patient look straight at you, and observe the direction of his gaze. Is there a deviation of one eye—a strabismus? In what direction does this deviation occur? Exodeviation describes a turned out eye; esodeviation describes a turned in eye. Observe if there is an involuntary jerking of the eye, known as a *nystagmus.*

The direction of the gaze of the eye is controlled by six muscles. These muscles are under the control of three cranial nerves. The six muscles are the two oblique (superior and inferior) and the four rectus muscles (superior, medial, lateral, and inferior). There are three cranial nerves that innervate or control these muscles. The fourth cranial (trochlear) nerve controls the superior oblique muscle and therefore downward nasal movement. The sixth cranial (abducens) nerve controls the lateral rectus muscle and therefore lateral deviation. The third cranial (oculomotor) nerve controls all other movements of the eye.

Muscles do not work independently. When the muscle is contracting (turning the eye toward that muscle), its antagonist—the one that produces the opposite effect—is relaxing.

Several tests are needed to evaluate the muscle function of the two eyes. First, have the patient look at your finger or a light in the straight ahead position. Occlude the right eye while watching the left eye. If the left eye moves, a strabismus is present. If the left eye does not move, it was fixing properly before the occluder was placed over the right eye. Now remove the occluder, wait a moment, and repeat the procedure, this time occluding the left eye. If neither eye moves, the eyes are probably straight. This test is called the cover-uncover test.

Next occlude the right eye and move the occluder to the left eye without allowing both eyes to be uncovered. Watch the eye that is being uncovered. If either eye moves, a phoria is present. This test

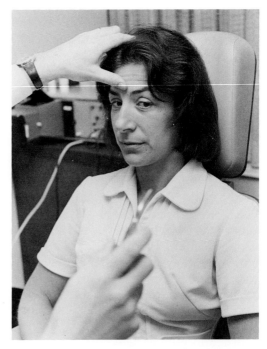

Figure 9-1. *Check muscle for gaze deviation. (Photo courtesy of Frank Flanagin, Associated Retinal Consultants, Detroit.)*

is called the cover test. It will also demonstrate an intermittent strabismus that may have been missed on the cover-uncover test.

Next examine the six major positions in which the eye moves. Take your finger and hold it to the person's left, asking him to look at your finger (Fig. 9-1). You are now testing the left gaze and the left lateral rectus and the right medial rectus muscles. Then move your finger to the right, then up and right, then up and left, then down and right, and lastly down and left. This test will demonstrate muscle paralysis. (For further testing and evaluation, see Chap. 4.)

REFLEXES

Next the corneal reflex may be tested. Generally we do not test this reflex if the patient is conscious and if we are aware that he has the blink reflex. If the test is to be done, take a piece of cotton such as a cotton ball and brush lightly over the cornea (the clear covering over the colored part of the eye). If the

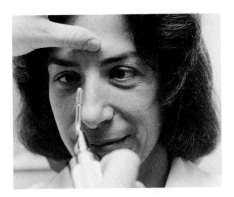

Figure 9-2. *Check for accommodation by moving object toward nose. (Photo courtesy of Frank Flanagin, Associated Retinal Consultants, Detroit.)*

patient blinks, the ophthalmic branch of the fifth cranial (trigeminal) nerve is intact.

Check the pupil for a light reflex, this reflex is controlled by the third cranial (oculomotor) nerve. Have the patient look at you and shine a flashlight into the right pupil. The constriction of the pupil is a direct response to your shining the flashlight into that eye. Look at the left pupil (while the light is directed into the right eye); constriction of the left pupil as a result of the light shining in the right pupil is known as a *consensual response.* The constriction of both pupils is a normal response to direct light. Lesions of the optic or oculomotor cranial nerves on the side being tested can cause a loss of the direct light reflex. Lesions of the optic nerve on the side being tested or to lesions of the oculomotor nerve on the opposite side can result in loss of the consensual light reflex.

ACCOMMODATION

Observe your patient for accommodation. Take your index finger and ask the patient to watch your finger. Hold your finger approximately eight inches from his nose. Move your index finger in toward his nose (Fig. 9-2). You will note that, as the patient watches your finger, his eyes should converge and his pupils constrict equally. When he stops accommodating, the pupils will begin to enlarge. This same test will demonstrate ability to converge the eyes when looking at near objects. Some people are able to converge better than others, and this may be important in evaluating muscle abnormalities. This is a test for the *accommodation–convergence reflex.* Lack of this reflex indicates a disorder of the third cranial nerve.

VISUAL EXAMINATION

ACUITY

Next examine the eye for visual acuity. This will be testing the second cranial (optic) nerve. The Snellen chart is generally one of the simpler tools used to record vision. The patient should be 20 feet from the chart and read the line that he feels he sees most clearly. If he reads this line perfectly, he should be asked to read the next line. For example, if the patient is asked to read the 20/50 line and if two letters are incorrectly viewed, you can record 20/50-2. This means that at 20 feet, the patient can read approximately what the "normal eye" can read at 50 feet. Legal blindness is defined as vision of 20/200 or less, which indicates that the patient can not read letters smaller than the 20/200 line on the Snellen chart.

Another method of assessing visual acuity is to hold your fingers in front of the patient's eyes and ask him to count the number of fingers you are holding up or that they can see. This is referred to as *count fingers* (C.F.) vision, and is recorded on the chart in that way. Some people may not be able to count fingers but can see a hand moving. This is recorded as "H. M. in O. D." or "H. M. in O. S."

Light perception is an indication of a viable retina. If a patient is blind (not able to see) but responds to a light flashed in his eye, he is said to have light perception. The flashlight should be directed into each pupil and recorded as "L. P. in O. D." or "no light perception in O. D."

Near vision can be checked by using a chart designed for testing near vision. There are many, but an example is the Jaeger chart. It is held 14 inches from the eye. The patient reads the smallest size printed paragraph that is readable to him. This is recorded on a scale standardized for measuring vision when using this chart. The scale is specifically for this chart and is not transferable from one type of near vision chart to another.

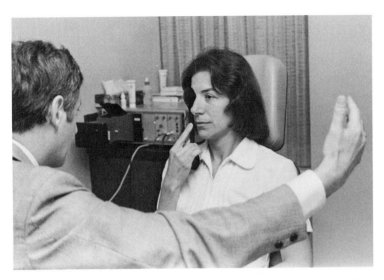

Figure 9-3. *Confrontation test. Right eye of patient is covered with eye occluder. Examiner is testing the left peripheral field of the patient's left eye. (Photo courtesy of Frank Flanagin, Associated Retinal Consultants, Detroit.)*

VISUAL FIELDS

Next, the patient is examined for visual fields. (See Perimetry, p. 254.) A confrontation test, although a crude method of testing peripheral vision, may be utilized rather than perimetry (see Fig. 9-3). In a confrontation test, the examiner and the patient sit facing one another, their knees almost touching. The examiner asks the patient to look directly into his eyes and to remain doing this throughout the test. The patient is told that when he views the examiner's finger coming into his line of vision he should indicate this immediately. The examiner then covers his own right eye and the patient covers his left eye with an occluder. The examiner then takes his finger and brings it from the nonseeing area into the patient's line of vision. His finger must be on a plane equidistant between patient and examiner. Various radii are examined. Both examiner and patient then occlude the opposite eye and the same procedure is repeated. Both examiner and patient should see the finger at approximately the same time. This test presupposes that the examiner has good peripheral vision. To test visual fields the patient must be alert, not medicated, and able to focus on the examiner's eyes. If reaction or response time is interfered with by sedation, the visual fields are not accurate.

PRESSURE

A tonometry exam may be performed to evaluate for increased intraocular pressure and the possibility of glaucoma. (See Testing for Glaucoma, p. 256.)

RETINA

A funduscopic examination is then performed to view the retina. (See Ophthalmoscope, p. 152.)

ASSESSMENT OF CHILDREN

Examining children for accurate findings in their visual abilities can be difficult. All school systems utilize some visual screening program. Most of these examine for near and far visual acuity and test for strabismus or phorias. There are numerous examinations available, and most important is the child's cooperation and ability to understand directions.

Examining the young child can be difficult. For the very young children, puppets are placed over an occluder, and the child is told to watch the puppet. At this point the examiner has the child's attention and tries visually to note any eye deviation. The cover–uncover test can be utilized by having the child interested in watching the puppet.

The illiterate E is frequently utilized to test the visual acuity of young children. Generally children are told that it is a table and to point in the direction that the legs point. The examiner shows the child where the legs are and says now these legs are pointing up, while pointing upward. The examiner then asks where do you see the legs on this table, pointing to the next E. This is one of the more popular visual acuity tests.

The better a story teller one is and the better the rapport one has with children, the easier one finds screening the very young child. With an alert clinician, both mother and child can be put to ease and a successful examination completed.

INSTRUMENTATION TECHNIQUES

VISUAL ASSESSMENT

Industry demands a rapid screening procedure for visual function— an important part of pre-employment physicals, and helpful when an employee chooses to transfer from one position to another. The safety of employees is a concern of industry. The need to protect employees and prevent avoidable accidents has initiated visual screening examinations.

An examination that is frequently used involves the Telebinocular test, which determines fusion, muscle coordination, far vision, near vision, color discrimination, depth perception, and peripheral visual fields. Many manufacturers produce Telebinoculars with various cards for visual screening. The Keystone tests are simply examples of the visual screening examinations that are available.

If an employee wears glasses, he should be permitted to wear them when performing the visual screening tests, to simulate the manner in which he would be viewing "the world" at work.

The employee is seated looking into the Telebinocular, and given a series of 15 tests (see Fig. 9–4). The first card tests vertical muscle balance at a far point. The examiner asks the patient what he sees. He'll indicate a red ball and a yellow line. The examiner then asks where the yellow line is in relation to the red ball. The patient may respond by saying it passes through the red ball. The line should touch some area of the red ball. If the patient has difficulty with this examination, his glasses should be examined to see if they are bent or have been worn "askew." The employee who cannot pass this examination likely would not be safe around heavy equipment or near moving cranes, as he would likely have intermittent diplopia and see double.

The second card is a test for horizontal imbalance at a far point. The card has an arrow and numbers from 1 through 15. The patient is asked at what number or between what numbers does the arrow come to rest. In order to pass this test within the normal range the employee should view the arrow between 7 and 11. If the arrow is seen outside this range the viewee may have a phoria, and have difficulty using both eyes together.

The third card is to test fusion at a far point. The patient is asked what he sees on the card. He will indicate the number of balls that he views on the card. He may see two, three, or four balls. Three balls indicate that the eyes are fusing for distance vision.

The next card is a test of distance visual acuity, of both eyes. The examiner tells the employees that in this picture there is a bridge with various signs. In each sign there are five diamonds. In each sign, one of these five diamonds has a black dot. Indicate the location of the dot in each sign starting with number 1. The

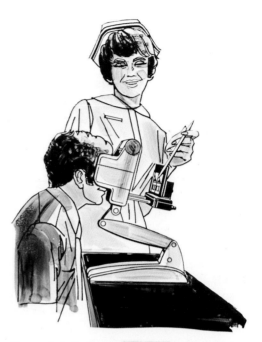

Figure 9–4. *Patient at Telebinocular.*

dot will be in the top, right, left, or bottom diamond. Good distance vision is important to comfortable vision and, depending on the job being applied for, an acceptable standard of vision may be indicated.

The fifth card tests far vision with the right eye. However, both eyes are used. The dots to be seen are only on the right side of the card. Hence, the right eye is being examined.

On the sixth card, far vision of the left eye is examined. This is a similar card with the dots being on the left side of the card.

The seventh card examines depth perception at a far point. In the first line you see a star, a square, a cross, a heart, and a ball. Which one stands out to you? The employee will answer. Then tell him to go through each line, naming the most prominent object. The percentage of stereopsis represented is from 10 to 65. To operate heavy equipment safely, it is felt that 50 percent stereoscopic ability is satisfactory. Depth perception is important for test drivers, the drivers of all vehicles, operators of heavy equipment, operators of equipment where accidents could cause serious injuries (e.g., large saws or heavy presses).

The eighth card examines for severe deficits in color vision discrimination. The examiner asks the employee to indicate the number in the three circles—top, lower left, and lower right.

The ninth card examines for mild color vision discrimination. The examiner asks the employee to indicate the number in each circle—top, lower left, and lower right. Good color discrimination is necessary for pilots, railroad crews, or anyone involved with multiple colors, such as installers of telephone wires. Aesthetic and good color discrimination is necessary for buyers with large department stores, interior decorators, those employed in home improvement businesses, and designers of automobiles.

The far-vision testing is now completed. Next the near vision is examined. Near vision is essential for engineers, accountants, secretaries, and those who read for pleasure.

The tenth card examines vertical muscle balance at a near point. Indicate where the yellow line is in relation to the red ball (same as the first card).

The eleventh card examines lateral muscle balance at a near point. Indicate where the arrow is pointing (same as second card).

The twelfth card examines fusion at a near object. The examiner asks how many balls the applicant sees (same as third card).

The thirteenth card tests for near vision bilaterally. The examiner tells the employee that there are 22 small circles comprising one larger circle. Each of these 22 circles are identified as having lines, dots, or as plain. Beginning with the first circle, indicate whether it has lines, dots, or is plain.

The fourteenth card is for near vision of the right eye and the fifteenth card is for near vision of the left eye (both tests same for bilateral near vision).

At this point visual fields are tested. Ask the employee to view the white dot behind the picture holder on the Telebinocular. Remind him to keep viewing the white dot at all times but to indicate when he sees the white ball coming into his side vision while looking straight ahead at the white area behind the picture holder. The arc is then swung slowly into the patient's line of vision. Each side is tested three times. The field is marked as read on the perimeter arm when the employee indicates he sees the white marker coming into view.

This completes the visual screening examination. If abnormal findings appear, the individual is referred to an ophthalmologist for further evaluation. The total examination takes approximately 50 minutes to administer. Figure 9–5 shows a record (A) with the normal values to be superimposed on a transparency (B).

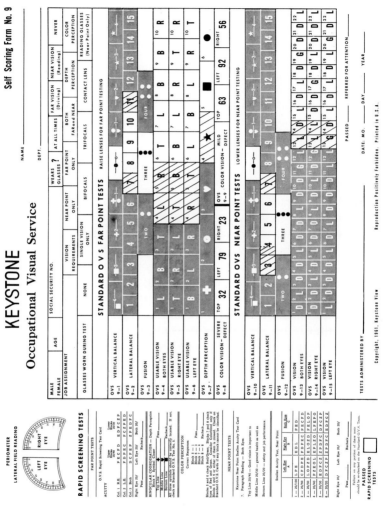

Figure 9–5. A. Record for employee's chart.

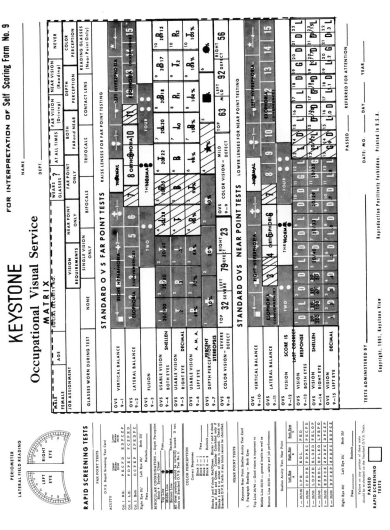

Figure 9-5 (continued). *B. Overlay for correction of test.*

VISUAL FIELD TESTING

Perimetry

Perimetry is the technique of testing the function of the peripheral retina, or more simply, the field of vision. The peripheral retina is not capable of fine discrimination and, therefore, the testing methods do not use objects requiring fine discrimination.

Many methods have been developed to test the sensitivity of the peripheral field, but the most widely used clinical technique involves moving a target from outside the field toward the fixation point.

There are two basic tests: central fields and peripheral fields. Central fields are performed on a flat screen, which is approximately one meter square. It is placed one meter (1000 mm) from the patient, and at this distance subtends about 50° of an arc (25° to each side of fixation) on the retina. Peripheral fields are performed on an instrument with a curved surface in the shape of one-half of a sphere having a radius of 330 mm (Fig. 9–6). The patient is positioned so that the eye being tested is at the center of the sphere. In each instance, the testing targets are round lights or discs. The targets are sized in millimeters and the common sizes are 1 mm, 2 mm, 3 mm, 5 mm, and 10 mm. White targets are always used, but colored targets are helpful in certain diseases, and may be used during the same examination. In recording, size and type of target should be designated. Thus, "3/1000 white" should indicate that a central field had been performed at 1000 mm with a 3 mm white target.

It is important that certain facts be noted on the field chart: (1) name, (2) date, (3) vision, (4) pupil size, (5) test object size, (6) distance, and (7) test object color.

To perform a field test properly, it is most important to have the patient seated comfortably. Because each eye is tested separately, the opposite eye must be covered. The patient is asked to look at the center point of fixation on whatever instrument is being used. It is essential that the patient look only at the central fixation point during the test, or the test will be inaccurate. The examiner must constantly monitor the patient to be sure that his fixation is not wandering. The target is then moved from outside the field of view into the field on a radial line toward the fixation point. The target is moved at a leisurely but constant pace until it reaches the center of fixation. It is then removed, taken outside the field, and started on a new radius. Usually about 12 to 18 radii are

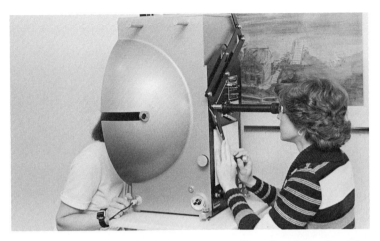

Figure 9–6. *Perimetry. Goldman perimeter. Examiner is on the right. Movement of the lever in her right hand moves the target light inside the sphere. (Photo courtesy of Frank Flanagin, Associated Retinal Consultants, Detroit.)*

measured. The patient is asked to indicate the moment he sees the target as it is brought into the field of view. This point is marked in each radius tested. As the target is moved toward fixation, the patient is asked to indicate if the target dims or disappears. If the patient does describe such an occurrence, it may indicate a neurologic defect in either the nerve supply to the eye or in the retina. This is called a *scotoma.* The target should be placed within the scotoma and moved outward from the center of the scotoma in all directions until the outlines of the scotoma have been delineated. The rule is to move the target from a non-seeing area to a seeing area.

The optic disc will always be able to be outlined in an accurate central field. This lies between 12° to 20° temporal to fixation and will be an oval about 15° in height in the normal eye.

After the examiner has completed the examination, the findings are then transferred to a chart, which is kept as a permanent part of the record (See Figs. 9–7 and 9–8).

Confrontation Test

The confrontation test is a simple but crude method of testing visual fields. The examiner sits facing the patient at approximately one meter distance. Each eye is tested individually, so the opposite eye must be covered. For example, the examiner covers his

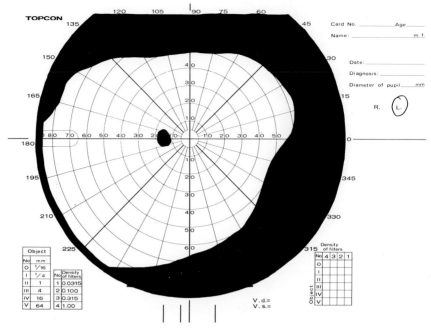

Figure 9–7. *Normal peripheral visual field, left eye.*

own left eye and the patient, his right eye. The point of fixation should be the eyes coming in direct contact. Remember the rule of moving from the nonseeing to the seeing area. The target, usually the examiner's finger, is moved in from the outside into the field of vision. The examiner's hand is kept equally distant between the patient and examiner. The examiner's field of vision is assumed normal and is therefore the standard against which the patient's field is compared. Multiple radii are tested. Each eye is examined using this method. A rough sketch or a description of the findings is placed on the patient's chart.

TESTING FOR GLAUCOMA

The Schiøtz tonometer is the most commonly used instrument to measure the intraocular pressure; hence it is invaluable in the diagnosis of glaucoma.

The patient must sit in a reclining chair or lie supine, looking at the ceiling. Each eye being examined is first anesthetized by instilling into the conjunctival sac an anesthetic agent, such as one

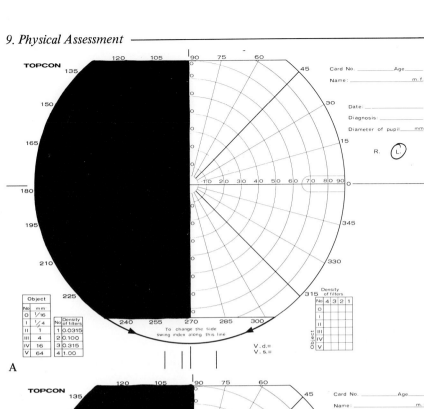

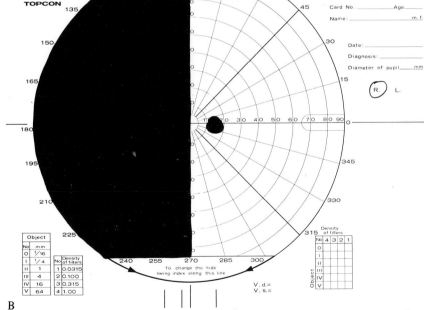

Figure 9–8. *Abnormal visual fields. Left homonymous hemianopsia caused by lesion in the right optic tract and demonstrating a peripheral field defect. A. Left half of the left visual field. B. Left half of the right visual field.*

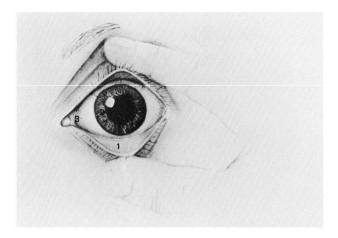

Figure 9–9. *Method of holding lids for placement of Schiøtz tonometer on cornea.*

or two drops of tetracaine hydrochloride 0.5% or propanacaine hydrochloride 1%.

An important part of the tonometry exam is that the patient fixate steadily on a specific spot on the ceiling. If he cannot do this, he should be asked to hold his arm in extension toward the ceiling. He is then told to look at his thumb; even a blind person will be able to sense where his thumb is and in most instances, be able to maintain steady fixation.

The tonometer should be held in the examiner's right hand (or left for left-handed individuals) and the other hand used to expose the cornea by retracting the upper and lower lids without exerting pressure on the globe (Fig. 9–9).

It is necessary for the surface of the cornea to be parallel to the floor. The most important thing is that the tonometer be in a vertical position in the center of the cornea.

The tonometer is then gently placed vertically on the apex of the cornea (Fig. 9–10).

The reading is taken from the scale of the tonometer, and the calculation is determined by referring to a Schiøtz scale. A normal reading is 12 to 22 mm Hg. The reading is recorded as T.O.D. = 14 Schiøtz (5.5 gm). Therefore, the reading of the right eye with the 5.5 gm weight attached to the tonometer is 14 and would be within the normal limits.

After taking the reading in each eye, the nurse should remind the patient that the cornea has been anesthetized by the eyedrop

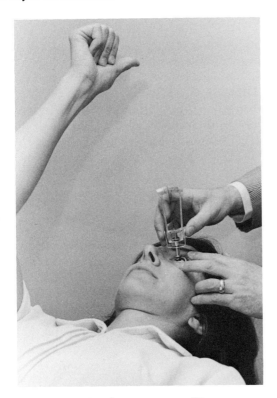

Figure 9–10. *Schiøtz tonometry. (Photo courtesy of Frank Flanagin, Associated Retinal Consultants, Detroit.)*

instilled before performing the procedure. It is important that the patient does not rub his eye as he may inadvertently scratch the cornea. If this procedure is used as a screening mechanism for an employee, he should not be permitted to be around machinery until the effects of the anesthetic have worn off, because a foreign body might lodge in his eye and he would be unaware of its presence.

The Schiøtz tonometer has various weights. The 5.5 gm weight is permanently attached to the tonometer. The other three weights are 7.5, 10, and 15. The 5.5 gm weight is adequate to test pressures within the normal range. If the intraocular pressure is elevated, more weight must be placed on the instrument, to indent the cornea enough to register on the scale. One chooses the weight that gives a reading between 3 and 7 on the scale, because the instrument functions most accurately within this range. The scale is marked from 0 to 20. The higher the scale registers, the lower the pressure—the greater the indentation the softer the eye. There is a different conversion table for each weight.

The Schiøtz tonometer can be wiped off with a commercially prepared solution for cleaning the instrument. An older method is to soak the instrument in ether for 20 minutes, and then rinse it with sterile distilled water. Another method is to permit the tonometer to stand in alcohol for 20 minutes, and then rinse it with sterile distilled water before reusing it on the next patient. It is essential to have the tonometer dry before using it, as alcohol or ether will cause a mild but uncomfortable corneal epithelial burn.

OPHTHALMOSCOPY

The instrument used to view the interior of the eye is called the ophthalmoscope. There are two techniques for ophthalmoscopy, direct and indirect.

Direct Ophthalmoscope

The direct ophthalmoscope is the one used most frequently in the United States. A direct ophthalmoscope is a cylinder, about two-thirds the size of a flashlight, with a round or oval disc attached to one end. The cylinder carries flashlight batteries. The disc contains a small hole on the side away from the handle.

Within the disc is a light, which is directed out one side of the hole, and a disc containing various lenses the size of the hole. The examiner looks through the hole and thus is looking along the beam of light exiting from the other side of the hole. He directs the light into the patient's pupil and, by rotating the lenses, can bring the patient's retina into focus. The image is erect, that is, exactly the way it would look if you could look through the pupil with the naked eye, but it is magnified about 15 times.

The examiner can perform ophthalmoscopy with or without glasses. If he normally wears corrective lenses, the ophthalmoscopic lens will compensate for both the patient's and the examiner's refractive error.

The instrument is held close to the examiner's eye and he positions himself close to the patient's pupil (see Fig. 7–5). The nearer the examiner is to the patient the greater are his chances of viewing the fundus. Examination of the fundus is best carried out in a dark room with the patient's pupils dilated. The retina can be seen without dilatation of the pupil, but it is like viewing a room through a keyhole rather than a picture window. Therefore, we feel that for adequate evaluation of the retina, dilatation of the pupil is essential.

The patient should be in a sitting position, facing the examiner. The examiner may sit or stand as preferred. The examiner should always be on the same side as the eye being examined. If the examiner does not have a visual disability, he will use his right eye to view the patient's right eye.

The patient is told to look straight ahead at an object approximately six inches above the examiner's shoulder.

To begin examining the patient's eye, hold the ophthalmoscope approximately 15 inches from his eye. Rotate the lens to 0 while directing the ray of light into the patient's eye. In the normal eye, the pupil will be filled with a reddish-yellow light, known as the *red fundus reflex*. This red color is the result of the reflection of light off the blood-filled choroid.

With the opthalmoscope set at 0, move in toward the eye without losing the fundus reflex. The closer the examiner can get to the patient's eye, the wider his field of view will be. Once that distance has been reached, the fundus is brought into focus by rotating the ophthalmoscope dial. Higher minus lenses (the red numbers on the dial) are needed for myopic persons, and higher plus lenses (the black numbers) for people with hyperopia.

If the patient has been looking straight ahead approximately six inches above your shoulder, you should be viewing his optic disc. Check the size of the physiologic cup as well as shape and color of the disc. Note how the vessels branch out of the cup.

The ratio of the diameter of the arteries to veins will be approximately 3:5. The arteries appear more straight, smaller in diameter, and a brighter shade of red. The veins are dark red, wider in diameter, and appear more tortuous (Fig. 9–11).

The entire fundus should be examined in an orderly manner. The fundus is generally divided vertically into temporal and nasal segments, each of these being examined superiorly and inferiorly. The fundus is referred to as a clock—the disc being the center, superior being 12, inferior being 6, temporal 9, and nasal 3 (on right eye). In the left eye 9 is nasal and 3 is temporal. The findings can be recorded by a sketch or in a descriptive paragraph.

To begin, follow the vessels upward. Note any discoloration, abnormal caliber of vessels, or vessel crossings. Watch for markings and changes in color or pigmentation of the fundus. Follow the same procedure for all four quadrants. All areas of each quadrant must be examined as far into the periphery as possible.

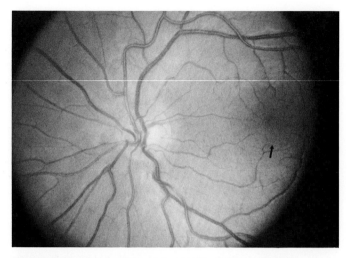

Figure 9-11. *Normal disc and macula. Arrow points to macula. Vessels are coming out of disc. (Photo courtesy of Frank Flanagin, Associated Retinal Consultants, Detroit.)*

Usually the macula is examined last because it is more sensitive to light than the rest of the retina and it will accommodate to the brightness while the periphery is being examined. The macula will be in view if the patient looks straight into the light.

The macula is a roughly oval area, darker than the rest of the fundus because of increased pigment, and easily recognized because there are no blood vessels at its center.

It is about 1½ disc diameters wide and 1 disc diameter high (1 disc diameter equals the width of the optic disc). The center of the macula is approximately 1½ disc diameters temporal to the temporal edge of disc. This spot is called the *fovea* and in the normal eye is seen as a yellowish dot.

Indirect Ophthalmoscope

The indirect ophthalmoscope, as used in the United States, is a binocular head-mounted instrument. Monocular hand-held instruments are also available. The indirect ophthalmoscope has a much brighter light to illuminate the retina. The light is mounted above a small viewing box that aligns the examiner's eyes so that he can look down the light beam. The examiner's eyes should be about 30 inches from the patient's eyes. The retina is focused with a hand-held convex lens. The image is totally inverted, which

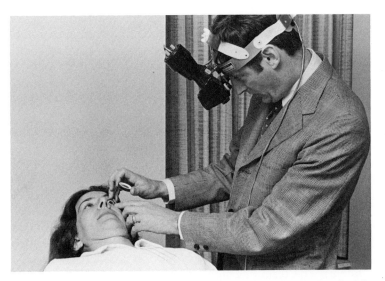

Figure 9-12. *Indirect ophthalmoscope in use. Lens in examiner's right hand focuses light through pupil. (Photo courtesy of Frank Flanagin, Associated Retinal Consultants, Detroit.)*

means that it would be like looking at a picture turned upside down. In addition, there is much less magnification, usually about three times.

Indirect ophthalmoscopic examinations are performed more easily if the patient is supine (Fig. 9-12). The pupil must be widely dilated; a cycloplegic combined with a mydriatic will give the best dilatation. The light is so bright that the pupil dilated with a mydriatic alone, no matter how widely dilated, will almost always partly constrict when the light strikes the eye. The light is directed into the patient's pupil from a distance of about 30 inches. The red reflex of the fundus is brought into view and the hand-held lens is then moved into the red reflex about midway between the patient and the examiner. The lens is then moved toward the patient's eye until the retina comes into sharp focus, which usually occurs about 3 or 4 inches from the eye. Focus is maintained by moving the hand-held lens forward and back. If a new area of the retina needs to be examined, the examiner's head and the lens must be moved in synchrony, always keeping the pupil, the lens, and the examiner's eye in a straight line.

The advantages of the indirect ophthalmoscope are that a greater field is obtained, and minor opacities, such as early cataract, do not obscure visualization so much. The result is a better appreciation of retinal diseases covering a wide area. The advantages of the direct ophthalmoscope are greater magnification and an upright image. Each instrument has its place and in fact complement each other in the total evaluation of retinal architecture and disease.

REFRACTION

Refraction is the term used in ophthalmology for the technique of neutralizing abnormal focusing power of the eye.

The eye that is in perfect focus at distance when the accommodation is completely relaxed is said to be normal. "Distance" is any point beyond 20 feet, because light rays entering the eye from beyond 20 feet are essentially parallel. This condition is called *emmetropia,* and when it exists an object in the distance is focused precisely on the retina. If a distance object is focused in front of the retina in a relaxed eye, the condition is called *myopia* (nearsightedness). The term *nearsightedness* has been used because the image can be moved farther back in the eye by moving the object closer to the eye. The image can also be moved back by placing concave (minus) lenses in front of the eye. If a distance object cannot be brought to focus within the eye by the eye's relaxed lens system (i.e., if the distance object would be focused farther back than the retina if the posterior wall of the eye were not present), the condition is called *hyperopia* or *farsightedness.* The condition cannot be resolved by moving the object farther away because the object is already in the distance. The condition can be resolved by placing convex (plus) lenses in front of the eye.

Thus, by placing plus lenses in front of a hyperopic eye or minus lenses in front of a myopic eye, the abnormal eye focus can be neutralized.

In addition to the hyperopic or myopic refractive error, most people also have an *astigmatic error* or *astigmatism.* The focusing power of simple myopia or hyperopia is the same in each meridian, whereas the focusing power in astigmatism is different in each meridian. The best way to understand this is to think of the surface of a simple lens as the surface of a mixing bowl and that of an astigmatic lens as the surface of a spoon. The bowl has meridians of equal curvature throughout. The spoon has a long curvature in one meridian, a short curvature 90° opposite to it, and varying amounts of curvature in between. In a much less pronounced fashion, this describes the difference in the lens systems of simple myopia or hyperopia and myopic astigmatism or hyperopic astigmatism.

The power of lenses and thus of refractive errors is designated in diopters. Dioptric power is measured by the following formula: D = 1/f, where D equals diopters and f equals the focal length of the lens in meters. Thus, if a lens focuses parallel light rays at 20 cm, dioptric power would be figured as follows:

$$D = \frac{1}{f} \quad (20 \text{ cm} = 0.2 \text{ meter})$$

$$D = \frac{1}{.2}$$

D = 5, or 5 diopters.

The technique for determining the refractive error is divided into two steps: objective and subjective. However, because the proper distance correction is the end point of this examination, the patient must have his accommodation relaxed before the examination begins. Most adults can relax their accommodation by staring into the distance. If there is a question as to whether accommodation is relaxed, a cycloplegic eyedrop should be used to paralyze the accommodation. Children have very strong accommodation and must receive cycloplegic drops to paralyze their focusing power. The objective determination of the eye's focusing power is accomplished with an instrument called a *retinoscope*. Using this instrument, the examiner directs a beam of light through the patient's pupil from a distance. The retinoscope light is moved across the pupil and the reflex is observed. If the reflex moves opposite to the movement of the retinoscope, minus lenses are added in front of the patient's eye, to move the focus out toward the examiner, and vice versa. If astigmatism is present, spherical lenses are used to neutralize one meridian, and cylindrical lenses are used to neutralize the meridian at right angles to the first.

When the proper combination of lenses has been placed before the patient's eye, the reflex does not change when the retinoscope is moved in any direction, and the endpoint of retinoscopy will have been achieved. However, the retinoscopist does not sit 20 feet from the patient. Thus, a correction in the retinoscopic findings must be made. Most examiners sit 26 inches (0.67 meter) in front of the patient. Since the lens needed to focus from distance to 0.67 meter is +1.50 D, this amount of lens power must be removed from the retinoscopic findings. If the retinoscopic findings show a result of +3.50 D, the true distance correction would be +2.00 D. If the findings show +0.50 D, the true correction would be –1.00 D. If astigmatism is present, the correction is always written with the sphere first, the cylinder power next, and the axis of the cylinder last. A cylinder axis is the direction that has no curve. For example, an oil barrel standing upright has a vertical axis. Horizontal axis is called 0° or 180°; vertical axis is called 90°. An astigmatic correction would be written in the following fashion:

+1.00 +1.25 X 45 [i.e., +1.00 sphere with an additional +1.25 cylinder at axis 45°]. These are other examples: –2.50 + 1.50 X 75, +2.00 (sphere only), –75 X 90 (cylinder only).

Any combination is possible. Most corrections fall between about +3.00 D and –3.00 D, and it is unusual for astigmatic error to be greater than 3.00 D. It is not usually necessary to prescribe corrections with greater accuracy than one quarter of a diopter. Therefore, lenses come in .25 D steps (e.g., +25, +50, +75, + 1.00, + 1.25, + 1.50, + 1.75, and so on). Occasionally a patient will be able to appreciate one-eighth diopter difference, but this is the smallest size that can be ordered.

Once the objective determination has been made, the patient is asked to read the eye chart, and slight amounts of plus and minus are added to both the spherical and cylindrical retinoscopic findings to achieve a subjective refinement of the retinoscopic findings. Often, the retinoscopic (objective) and subjective findings are identical. They are usually very close if a skilled retinoscopist has performed the examination. If there is great discrepancy, more weight is usually placed on the subjective findings. At the end of the subjective examination, the final distance correction is determined.

If the patient is under the age of 45 years he is usually able to use his distance correction with comfort at near. Over the age of 45, the accommodation power of the eye is reduced, so that the patient wearing his full-distance correction will need some plus lens to help him accommodate to the reading position. The first reading addition is usually about +.75 D or +1.00 D added to the distance correction. This is gradually increased so that by age of 50 years, about +1.50 D is needed, and by age 65 about +2.25 D is needed. Usually, little change is necessary after the age of 65 years.

The reading add may be prescribed in a bifocal or in a separate reading glass. But the amount is always added to the distance correction which is determined as described above. The patient must not have had cycloplegic drops instilled before the reading correction is tested because his own accommodation will be paralyzed and the reading correction will be made stronger than necessary. If cycloplegic drops have been used, the patient will have to return on another day for a postcycloplegic exam.

SELECTED READINGS

BOOKS

Bates, B. *A Guide to Physical Examination.* Philadelphia: Lippincott, 1974.

Keeney, A. H. *Ocular Examination Basis and Techniques.* St. Louis: Mosby, 1970.

Sana, J., and Judge, R. *Physical Appraisal Methods in Nursing Practice.* Boston: Little, Brown, 1975.

CHAPTER 10 —————————

SPECIAL NURSING MEASURES

EVERTING THE UPPER EYELID

Everting the upper eyelid permits the inspection of the superior palpebral conjunctiva. Foreign bodies frequently adhere in the horizontal sulcus that lies just superior to the lid margin, thus causing an irritation to the cornea.

Have the patient sit in a comfortable position. Instruct the patient to look down. (This relaxes the levator muscle, which is attached to the upper border of the tarsal plate.) It is important that the patient not squeeze his eyelids, as this causes a contraction of the orbicularis muscle and prevents the examiner from everting the eyelid. Gently grasp the eyelashes, and pull downward. Take an applicator and apply gentle pressure on the skin side of the eyelid pushing down on the upper tarsal border (Fig. 10–1). Then evert the eyelid by pulling the lashes up and rolling the lid over the applicator; as the lid is everted the applicator is removed and the lid is held in eversion by holding the eyelashes against the eyebrow (Fig. 10–2). The eyelid is now in eversion, and the upper conjunctival area can be examined or inspected. It is important for the patient to continue to look down throughout this examination. When the patient looks up, the eyelid will flip back and return to its normal position.

To examine the superior conjunctival fornix, a double everting technique is indicated.

Use the previous technique but use the applicator on skin side of lid and push downward to expose the superior fornix.

INSTILLATION OF EYE MEDICATION

EYEDROPS

Eyedrops are instilled for various purposes. They dilate the pupil, constrict the pupil, reduce inflammation, or anesthetize the conjunctiva and cornea.

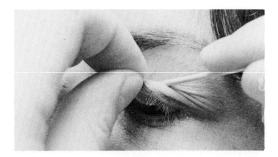

Figure 10–1. *To evert the eyelid, place the cotton applicator on skin side of the upper lid, grasp lashes, and lift. (Photo courtesy of Frank Flanagin, Associated Retinal Consultants, Detroit.)*

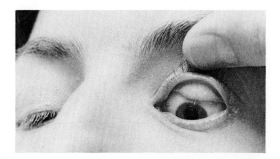

Figure 10–2. *Light pressure to eyelashes holds lid everted as long as patient continues to look down. (Photo courtesy of Frank Flanagin, Associated Retinal Consultants, Detroit.)*

There are three methods of instilling eyedrops:

1. Drop may be placed in the lower conjunctival sac.
2. Drop may be placed over the superior scleral area, thereby flowing downward over the cornea and pupil.
3. In a crying infant, a drop may be placed in the nasal canthus area. The lower lid is pulled down so that the drop rolls into the conjunctival sac.

If the lids are crusted, clean the eyelashes with a saline-soaked cotton ball before instilling the eyedrops. Secretions often adhere to the lashes and one must stroke downward (Fig. 10–3) and across

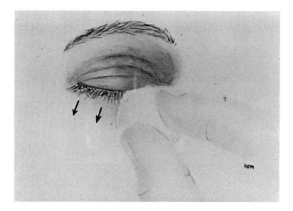

Figure 10–3. *Remove mucus crusting that adheres to the lashes by stroking downward.*

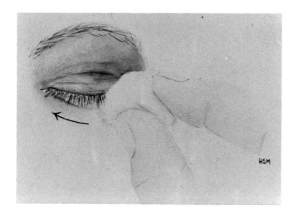

Figure 10–4. *To remove secretions wipe across eye from inner to outer canthus.*

(Fig. 10–4) to remove these secretions. At times the eyes have so much discharge they look "glued shut."

Technique

   FIRST METHOD. Position the patient in a horizontal supine position, or have the patient sit with his neck hyperextended, looking toward the ceiling.

   With the thumb or finger, pull down firmly on the lower lid, having the patient look upward. This relaxes the upper tarsal plate

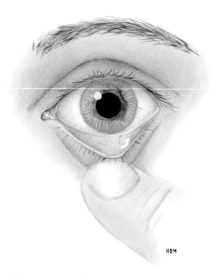

Figure 10–5. *Pulling down on lower lid to expose conjunctival sac.*

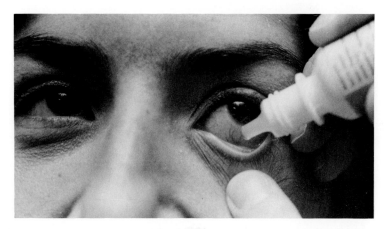

Figure 10–6. *Eyedrop installed in lower conjunctival sac. (Photo courtesy of Frank Flanagin, Associated Retinal Consultants, Detroit.)*

as it is retracted into the orbit and exposes the lower conjunctival sac (Fig. 10–5).

Place one drop of medication into the lower conjunctival sac (Fig. 10–6). Permit the patient to close his eye but not to squeeze. Wipe away excess tearing with a cotton ball or tissue. A two-by-

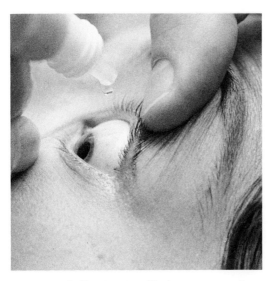

Figure 10-7. *Eyedrop instillation over superior scleral area. (Photo courtesy of Frank Flanagin, Associated Retinal Consultants, Detroit.)*

two inch gauze square should not be used because it may scratch the cornea. Also, some strands of the gauze could adhere to the lashes causing irritation or scratching of the cornea when the eyelid is opened.

If more than one drop is to be instilled, permit the patient to close his eye between drops to permit the medication to be absorbed. Patients do blink or close their eyes as a reflex action. Permitting them to do this makes it easier in holding the eye open for the next drop.

SECOND METHOD. To permit the drop to flow down over the cornea and pupil, position the patient in a Fowler's or semi-Fowler's position, with the neck slightly hyperextended (Fig. 10-7). With the thumb or the finger of one hand, firmly pull upward on the upper lid, permitting the lid to rest on the superior portion of the eye. (Do not permit your hand to slip, thus putting pressure on the globe of the eye.) Have the patient look down. Place one drop of medication on the superior area of the sclera. After instillation of the drop, permit the patient to close his eye, but not to squeeze. Wipe away any excess tearing with a cotton ball or tissue. (Again, two-by-two gauze squares should not be used because a stray strand may scratch or irritate the cornea.)

If more than one drop is to be instilled, permit the patient to close his eyes between drops. This permits the medication to be absorbed, and the patient to be more cooperative in holding his eye open for any succeeding drops.

THIRD METHOD. Have the infant held in supine position. Place one drop of medication in the nasal canthus area. Spread the lids thus permitting the eyedrop to roll into the conjunctival sac. After instilling the eyedrop, a slight amount of pressure should be placed on the inferior punctum area. In young children and some adults, when the eyelids are closed or they blink, the eyedrop is pushed by gravity and capillarity into the nasolacrimal duct, thus being absorbed into the systemic circulation. Medication is absorbed more readily from the nasal mucosa than the conjunctiva. Because children weigh much less than adults, the systemic effect of any absorbed medication is greater and can be dangerous. Sometimes adults complain of an unpleasant taste in their mouth after receiving eyedrops. This is a result of draining through the nasolacrimal duct. Pressure placed over the punctum after instillation of eyedrops will prevent this unpleasant sensation.

EYE OINTMENT

Place the patient in a supine position or sitting with neck hyperextended. Any secretions should be wiped from the eye and lashes with sterile normal saline swabs.

Instruct the patient to look up, and with your thumb or finger, pull down firmly on the conjunctival sac.

A quarter-inch ribbon of ointment deposited on the inner surface of the lid is probably sufficient. However, larger amounts of ointments will not cause harm. In fact, spreading ointment along the lid margin is an effective way of getting ointment into a crying infant's eye, since enough medication will work its way into the conjunctival sac.

In squeezing the medication into the lower conjunctival sac, avoid contaminating the tube by touching the eye or conjunctiva. Also, the cornea or conjunctiva could be irritated by touching the "eye" with the medication tube.

Following the application of the ointment, the eye may be closed. Advise the patient to refrain from squeezing. In the post-operative patient, squeezing the eye is to be avoided as it raises intraocular pressure and puts stress on the suture line.

Note: If mothers are applying ointment to a baby's eye, one should remind them to wash their hands before and after instillation of medication. We have found that some mothers rub their own eyes, thus causing dilatation of their pupils if a mydriatic eye medication has been used.

CLEANING EYE PROSTHESIS

The ophthalmic prosthesis or artificial eye is removed to clean it and irrigate the socket.

The prosthesis is removed by gently depressing the lower lid and exerting a small amount of pressure under the lower edge of the prosthesis. The prosthesis will then slip out of the orbit because the suction is broken.

If a suction cup is used, the procedure is the same: apply suction and move the prosthesis down over the lower lid (Fig. 10–8).

The prosthesis can be washed by using Ivory soap and water. It should be rinsed thoroughly and inserted wet. Having the prosthesis wet for reinsertion reduces the friction between the prosthesis and conjunctiva lining the orbit. This permits easier reinsertion.

The socket generally is clean. Since the prosthesis is a foreign object, it must be removed and cleaned daily. If patients neglect to do this, a slight discharge can occur. The orbital socket can be irrigated if the patient hangs over the sink, taking a small rubber syringe of water and directing it to the back of the socket, permitting it to roll out the temporal side of the orbit. The nurse may irrigate the orbit using a disposable syringe and basin (Fig. 10–9).

To replace the prosthesis wet reduces friction. The upper portion of the prosthesis is placed under the upper lid, the lower lid is pulled down, and the lower edge of the prosthesis slipped behind the lower lid. With finger or thumb, gently pull down on the lower lid and slide the prosthesis into place (Fig. 10–10). The patient will be taught to remove, clean, and reinsert his or her own prosthesis. A suction cup may or may not be used for removal or reinsertion of the prosthesis (Fig. 10–11).

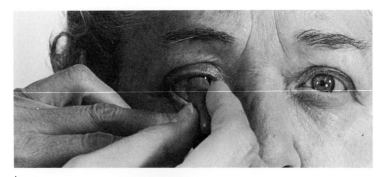

A

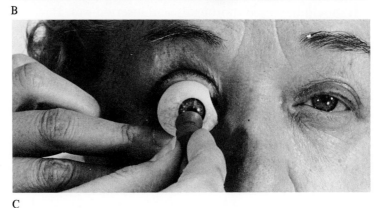

B

C

Figure 10-8. *A. The suction cup is placed on the prosthesis. Note left hand is depressing lower lid, while right hand is using suction cup. B. The pulling motion is out and down. The prosthesis is beginning to be slid over lower lid. C. Prosthesis as it is being slid from under the upper lid. (Photo courtesy of Csaba L. Martonyi, Department of Ophthalmology, The University of Michigan Medical School.)*

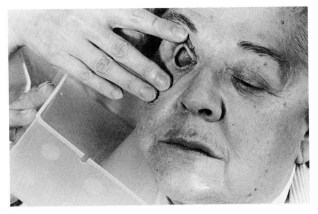

A

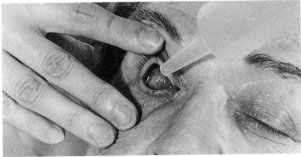

B

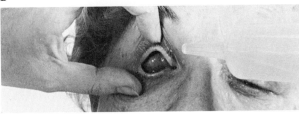

C

Figure 10-9. *A. Patient holds irrigating basin. B. Note eyelids can be held open by using index finger to hold upper lid against superior orbital rim and middle finger to depress lower lid against inferior orbital rim. Prosthesis has been removed. The convex appearance within the orbit is the anterior surface of the orbital implant covered by conjunctiva. C. Note eyelid could also be held open with index finger holding upper lid against superior orbital rim and thumb depressing lower lid against inferior orbital rim. (Photo courtesy of Csaba L. Martonyi, Department of Ophthalmology, The University of Michigan Medical School.)*

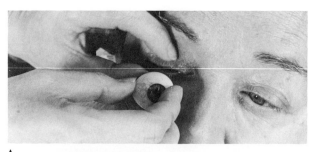

A

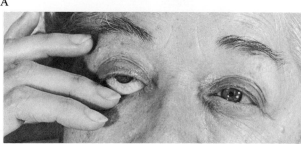

B

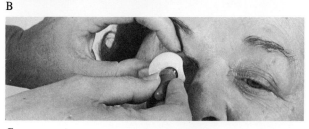

C

Figure 10-10. *A. Left hand separates lids while right hand holds prosthesis. B. Prosthesis is placed under upper lid first and is shown sliding over lower lid. C. Prosthesis is replaced with a suction cup. (Photo courtesy of Csaba L. Martonyi, Department of Ophthalmology, The University of Michigan Medical School.)*

EYE COMPRESSES

Warm compresses increase blood supply to a local area, while cold compresses constrict or decrease the blood supply to a local area.

There are many purposes for applying compresses: they aid in cleansing; they soothe; they decrease pain, ecchymosis, or edema;

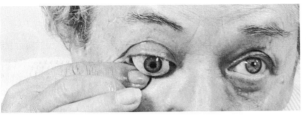

A

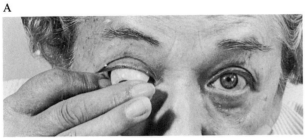

B

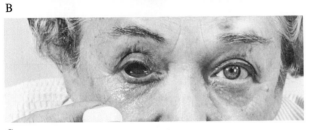

C

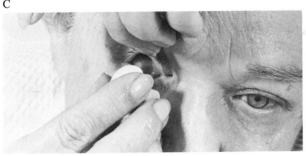

D

Figure 10–11. *A. Patient must learn to remove his or her own prosthesis by gently depressing lower lid. (Note suction is broken.) Prosthesis emerges over lower lid. B. Prosthesis is now sliding down from under upper lid. C. Prosthesis is successfully removed. D. Patient reinserts own prosthesis by holding upper lid against orbital rim and sliding superior edge of prosthesis in first. (Photo courtesy of Csaba L. Martonyi, Department of Ophthalmology, The University of Michigan Medical School.)*

they also can be used to reduce inflammation or cause vasoconstriction to a local area.

Compresses generally are ordered for 20 minutes, four times a day. The patient lies in the supine position, so that positioning will assist in holding the compress in place.

There are commercially prepared 4 X 4 compresses of sterile water and sterile normal saline available. These can be refrigerated or heated in a "warmer" prepared by the manufacturer.

The manner of obtaining a warm compress may vary in different institutions. If the agency does not utilize commercially prepared compresses, sterile 4 X 4s, a sterile basin, sterile solution, and sterile hemostats are needed. Solutions in their original container can be placed in a pan of water and warmed on the kitchen stove in the unit area. Some agencies simply place the sterile solution in a sink of extremely warm water.

The solution (warm or cold) is then poured into a basin, the squares are then put into the basin. The excess solution is removed by applying the hemostats to opposite corners, turning one clockwise and the other counterclockwise. When applied to the patient, warm compresses are covered with a sterile towel to maintain their warmth, while cold compresses remain open to the air to maintain cold.

When patients go home from the hospital they may use a clean washcloth as a compress. Warm tap water from the faucet is a "ready" solution. The washcloth can be quartered and a clean section of the cloth applied to the eye each time it is rewarmed by turning the faucet to the appropriate temperature.

IRRIGATION OF THE EYE

The most common reason for irrigating the eye is to remove a caustic substance such as a chemical. The essential principle to remember in removing a strong irritating chemical from the eye is that the chemical will continue to cause damage and destroy the cornea and damage the conjunctiva as long as it remains in contact with the eye.

Thus, the eye must be washed out copiously with tap water or any bland substance. Keep the lids open by firmly holding the upper lid against the superior orbital rim with your index or middle finger. Hold the lower lid against the inferior orbital rim with your thumb (Figs. 10–12 and 10–13). Holding the head slightly laterally, wash the eye copiously with tap water. If pos-

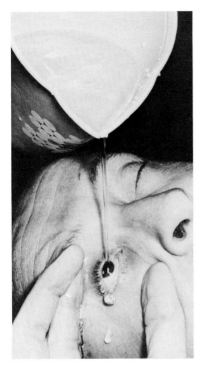

Figure 10–12. *Holding eyelid open and irrigating with water. (Photo courtesy of Csaba L. Martonyi, Department of Ophthalmology, The University of Michigan Medical School.)*

sible, the head could be held directly under the water faucet. Either way—using a glass or some type of container, or holding the eye directly under the water faucet—the patient finds the water uncomfortable, so a firm hold on lids is essential to assist the patient by removing the foreign substance. While it is not always possible, it is desirable to pour the water on the conjunctiva, permitting it to run over the cornea. Direct force of pouring water on the cornea causes discomfort and reflex blinking. You may have heard it said that the eye should be washed copiously for 20 minutes. This is not accurate. The eye should be washed until all caustic material has been removed. The aim is not dilution but removal of the foreign substance.

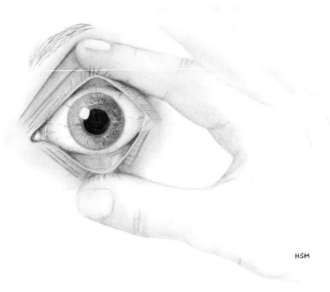

HSM

Figure 10–13. *Index finger holds lid against superior orbital rim while thumb holds lower lid against inferior orbital rim.*

After the eye has been thoroughly washed, the patient should be taken to a hospital emergency room or ophthalmologist's office for further treatment and diagnosis.

The first-aid treatment of removing the offending substance entirely from the eye is of prime importance. This thorough washing or irrigating could save a person's sight. Hesitancy, calling a physician, or rushing to a nearby hospital without first washing the eye could result in blindness.

Industries or laboratories where caustic materials are in use should have showers and water fountains that are to be used for immediate irrigation in the event of an accident. Nurses should see that these areas are clearly marked for emergency use.

EMERGENCY TREATMENT

Because emergency treatment of injuries is so important we feel that a special section of important points should be reiterated in this chapter and perhaps certain points clarified.

Nurses should always assess vision before beginning any emergency treatment. This may be having the patient read the line most visible on the Snellen chart. If there is a severe injury with a piece of sharp material protruding from the globe, you might then ask the patient to count your fingers. Visual assessment is an indication of the patient's vision after injury and is a protection against lawsuits for you and the institution. For example, after treatment, the patient may state that he could see when he entered the emergency room, but after treatment lost his eyesight. This simple but important rule is: "Hands off, until some sort of visual acuity is taken, be it ever so crude." This finding of course is written on the patient's record. Emergency room nurses, occupational health nurses, and school nurses must be alert to legal implications in treating the injured.

If the patient has a foreign body on the surface of the cornea, sclera, or conjunctiva and if it can be removed easily with a cotton applicator soaked in saline, this can be done. This object can usually safely be removed without further injury to the eye. For example if the substance is ground bits of glass, then the eye should be irrigated copiously with saline. The eyelid should be everted and a cotton applicator used to remove bits and slivers adhering under the palpebral conjunctiva. If the applicator is rolled do not roll it more than one complete turn so as not to grind particles of glass into the tissue of the eye particularly if any small slivers of glass adhere to the cornea.

If a foreign body is embedded in the cornea, sclera, or globe of the eye, a physician should treat the eye. Nurses should not try to remove an embedded foreign body. The rust rings that occur because of these injuries must be removed.

Eyelids or eyes that are bleeding generally should be permitted to bleed. Pressure applied to the lids of a severely injured eye could cause irretrievable damage by expressing ocular contents through a hidden scleral laceration. If someone can hold the bleeding lacerated upper lid against the orbit, pressure can be applied to stop bleeding. This is basically dangerous for the inexperienced person as the area is moist, the person nervous, and fingers slip, resulting in pressure to the globe of the eye. One *never* applies pressure to the globe of the eye.

If a foreign substance such as a chemical or alkali is splashed into the eye, the eye must be held open and thoroughly irrigated with water. This treatment is done immediately at the scene of the accident. The foreign substance continues to burn and destroy tissue as long as it remains in contact. Therefore, it is imperative for the eye to be copiously washed with water. Patients with chemical or alkali burns should always be treated by a physician after the emergency eyewash has been completed at the scene of the accident.

If the patient complains of discomfort and no injury is apparent a fluorescein strip may be used to demonstrate whether the cornea is abraded. Take a fluorescein strip, moisten with sterile saline, and touch it to the lower palpebral conjunctiva. Only a minute amount of fluorescein is necessary because it will spread over the entire cornea and conjunctiva. Any abraded area of the cornea will stain with fluorescein.

It is well for the nurse to remind patients seen in emergency rooms that, if their eye continues to feel uncomfortable in 24 hours, they should seek medical attention. Eyes that continue to be painful deserve further assessment and evaluation.

REMOVAL OF CONTACT LENSES

The cornea is normally lubricated by the tears, which are composed mainly of secretions from the lacrimal gland along with components from the meibomian glands and the sebaceous glands of the lids. The periodic blink permits the eyelids to spread this fluid over the corneal surface.

When contact lenses are worn, it is essential for a layer or film of "tears" to be between the contact lens and the cornea or sclera. The normal osmotic pressure of the cornea "tear film" is approximately the same as 0.9% sodium chloride solution. Therefore, the most satisfactory wetting agents are those that are isotonic with the normal tears. The person who wears contact lenses must maintain the cornea fluid film for the maintenance of corneal integrity.

Before removing a contact lens, this fluid film must be present or the epithelial or outermost layer of the cornea would be damaged. Therefore, if the eye appears dry (for example, in an unconscious patient after an accident), several drops of saline solution or a contact lens wetting solution should be instilled into the eye before attempting to remove a contact lens.

There are three types of contact lenses: the hard corneal lens, the soft contact lens, and the scleral lens. Each of these lenses requires a slightly different procedure for removal.

To remove contact lenses, have a patient lie in the supine position. In this way, the lens will not "pop out" onto the floor.

The lens will pop out and be retrievable from the edge of the eyelids.

To remove a hard corneal contact lens, stretch the upper lid temporally very tautly or tightly across the cornea with your thumb or middle finger. Then place your middle finger on the upper lid and the thumb of your other hand on the lower lid, gently moving the lids toward each other. This lid maneuver is done to trap the edge of the contact lens between the margins of the upper and lower eyelids. Do not press inward on the globe. The lids will trap the edge of the contact lens and break the suction, thus permitting the lens to pop out. If a suction cup is available, a hard lens may be removed in this way. The suction cup is applied to the hard lens and the lens slides easily off the cornea.

To remove the soft contact lens, elevate the eyelid superiorly holding it against the orbital rim. Gently place the thumb and index finger of the opposite hand on the contact lens, pinch the soft lens and it will pop off the cornea. This pinching motion is frightening at first, but extremely simple and nonirritating to the patient.

In removing the scleral lens, elevate the upper lid against the orbital bone, and pull down on the lower lid. Gently press on the upper lid. The scleral lens will move off the cornea. Spread the lids gently, and the lens will come free and can be removed.

The lens should be kept in a saline solution, the right lens being in a container marked *R* and the left lens being placed in a container marked *L*.

Lenses should be cleaned after each removal. Special cleaning solution is available, and directions for the care of lenses is vital for good hygiene and safety.

SELECTED READINGS

BOOKS

Henderson, V., and Nite, G. *Principles and Practice of Nursing* (6th ed.). New York: Macmillan, 1978. Pp. 806–812, 1321–1325.
Wolff, L. V., Weitzel, M., and Fuerst, E. V. *Fundamentals of Nursing* (6th ed.). Philadelphia: Lippincott, 1979. Pp. 356–359, 538–539, 621–623.

ARTICLES

Boyd-Monk, H. Taking a closer look at contact lenses. *Nursing '78,* pp. 38–43, Oct. 1978.

Boyd-Monk, H.   Screening for glaucoma. *Nursing '79,* pp. 42–45, Aug. 1979.

Gould, H.   How to remove contact lenses from comatose patients. *American Journal of Nursing* 76(9): 1483–1485, 1976.

Montague, R.   The pros and cons of hard and soft contact lenses. *Nursing Times* 72(26): 1018–1020, 1976.

Weinstock, F. J.   Tonometry screening glaucoma. *American Journal of Nursing* 73(4): 656–657, 1973.

Zucrik, M.   Care of an artificial eye. *American Journal of Nursing* 75(5): 835–836, 1975.

GLOSSARY

accommodation. The act of focusing the eye (i.e., of focusing the lens to the eye)

alpha-chymotrypsin. An enzyme that decreases the strength of the zonules that hold the lens

amblyopia. Decrease in vision without organic cause

angle-closure glaucoma. A pathologic state in which the intraocular pressure is elevated secondary to blockage of the aqueous outflow channels by bunching of the iris into the angle. This occurs in eyes predisposed to development of this condition by a narrowed anterior chamber angle

anterior chamber. The compartment of the eye bounded anteriorly by the cornea and posteriorly by the iris. It is filled with a watery fluid called aqueous

arcuate scotoma. A blind area in the field of vision extending in an arc fashion from the blind spot above or below the central point of fixation to the midline on the other side. These are typically early glaucoma field defects and are due to damage to the nerve fibers extending temporally from the optic nerve

Argyll Robertson pupil. A pathologic pupillary response, in which the pupil is miotic and can react to accommodation but does not react to light

astigmatism. A condition of the cornea in which the curvature of the cornea is different in some meridians from the curvature in other meridians

biconvex lens. A lens with a convex configuration to each side of its surface

blepharitis. A chronic infection of the glands and lash follicles along the lid margin

blepharochalasis. Relaxation of the lid tissue. A horizontal fold of excess tissue develops and may be severe enough to droop over the pupillary axis

cataract. Opacification of the lens

central visual fields. The test of the field of vision extending from fixation to approximately 30° to all sides of fixation. The test is usually performed by plotting the patient's ability to see small targets on a 1 meter square flat surface placed 1 meter from the patient's eye

chalazion. A cyst that results from a chronic infection of a meibomian gland

choroid. The thin vascular tissue layer that lies between the retina and the sclera on the innermost surface of the sclera

choroiditis. Inflammation of the choroid

ciliary body. A ring of vascular tissue and muscle that rests against the sclera just behind the peripheral extent of the iris. Its primary functions are to change lens focus and to produce aqueous fluid

ciliary flush. Engorgement of the episcleral vessels surrounding the cornea. This occurs in association with inflammation of the iris or ciliary body

confrontation test. A gross method of estimating the visual field by having the patient and the examiner face each other and using the examiner's field of vision as the normal

conjunctivitis. An infection of the conjunctiva

contact lens. A thin device of synthetic material, usually acrylic plastic, formed to fit snugly on the cornea

cornea. The transparent anterior wall of the eye through which light passes

count fingers. A visual designation used as an estimation of vision when the visual acuity is unreportable on standard charts

cryothermy. The freezing of tissue to form a therapeutic scar

cyclodialysis. An operation used to control glaucoma by separating a portion of the ciliary body from its attachment to the sclera

darkroom test. A provocative test for narrow angle glaucoma. The patient is kept in the dark for an hour. As the pupil dilates, blockage of aqueous outflow will occur if the entrance to the angle is narrow. A rise of 8 mm Hg is considered a positive test

diathermy. The heating of body tissue to form a therapeutic scar

dilating series. A series of cycloplegic and/or mydriatic eyedrops spaced at intervals usually of 5 to 10 minutes, the purpose of which is to dilate the pupil

diopter. The measure of the focusing power of a lens. The formula is as follows: $D = 1/f$, where D is power in diopters and f is the focal length of the lens in meters

diplopia. Double vision

direct ophthalmoscope. An instrument used to examine the inside of the eye. The configuration of the lens system is such that the examiner sees a real upright image

ecchymosis. Common "black eye"

ectropion. A condition in which the lid margin is everted away from the globe

electroretinography. A study measuring the retina's electric response to light stimulation

endophthalmitis. An inflammation of entire eye

entropion. A condition in which the lid margin is inverted so that the lashes rub on the globe

enucleation. Surgical removal of the eye

epiphora. Inability of the tear drainage system to handle the amount of tears produced. The result is excessive "tearing," and the usual cause is narrowing of the tear drainage channels

episcleritis. Inflammation of the episclera

erisiphake. An instrument used to grasp the lens by suction. It is used during cataract extraction

evisceration. The surgical technique of removing the inner contents of the eye, but leaving the sclera. It is felt that a better cosmetic result can be obtained by an evisceration than by an enucleation

external filtering procedure. A glaucoma operation, the purpose of which is to form an opening from the anterior chamber through the sclera into a pocket underneath the conjunctiva

extracapsular. A term applied to a technique of cataract surgery in which the capsule is ruptured and the cortex and nucleus are removed from the remnant of the capsule. The anterior capsule is usually removed and the posterior capsule remains

floaters. Any thickening portion of vitreous or deposit within the vitreous that will cast a shadow on the retina

fluorescein. A dye used topically or injected intravenously to assist in diagnosing pathology

glaucoma. A condition in which the intraocular pressure has become elevated sufficiently that it has caused structural or functional damage to the eye. The term is also applied when the pressure is elevated enough to cause structural damage even though the damage has not occurred, or when pressure can be controlled only by medication

gonioscopy. A technique of examining the anterior chamber angle

goniotomy. An operation for treatment of congenital glaucoma

gray line. A thin grayish-white line that runs along the surface of the lid margin. Its importance lies in its being a surgical landmark that designates the cleavage plane within the lid, splitting the posterior part (including conjunctiva and tarsus) from the anterior part (including orbicularis muscle and skin)

histoplasmosis. A fungal disease with ophthalmologic importance in that it forms a triad of retinal findings: punched out white peripheral retinal scars, submacular hemorrhage and scarring, and peripapillary atrophy

hordeolum (stye). An infection of the glands of Moll or Zeis

Horner's syndrome. A syndrome of abnormalities occurring within and around the eye, caused by paralysis of the cervical sympathetic nerve supply. The findings include ptosis, myosis, pseudo enophthalmos (a sinking of the eyeball) and anhidrosis of the face, all of the same side

hyperopia. A condition in which the relaxed lens of the eye is not powerful enough to focus parallel light rays (i.e., light rays from a distant object) onto the retina

hyphema. A condition caused by blood in the anterior chamber, producing a grossly visible level of blood

hypopyon. A condition caused by enough inflammatory cells present in the anterior chamber that a grossly visible level of white material is present

indirect ophthalmoscope. An instrument that provides a totally inverted image of the retina

internal filtering procedure. A surgical procedure for glaucoma that fashions a pathway of drainage from the anterior chamber to another chamber of the eye, usually the suprachoroidal space

intracapsular. A term applied to cataract removal without rupturing the lens capsule

intraocular lens implant. A small plastic lens placed within the eye following removal of the cataractous lens

intraocular pressure. The pressure above atmospheric pressure of the intra-ocular contents upon the surface of the eyeball expressed in millimeters of mercury (the normal is between 11 and 21 mm Hg)

iridectomy. The surgical procedure for removal of a section of the iris

iridodialysis. A condition in which the iris has been torn at its insertion into the sclera. The name applies whether the tear is very small or very large

iris. A curtain-like tissue that forms the posterior wall of the anterior chamber and rides on the surface of the lens. It is the iris that gives the eye its color

iritis. An inflammation of the iris

keratitis. An inflammation of the cornea

keratoconus. A condition in which the central cornea develops a noninflam-matory conical protrusion

keratoplasty. Any surgical procedure dealing with improving corneal clarity by removal or reduction of corneal scarring. In its narrow sense, the term usually applies to corneal grafting procedures

laceration. A torn, uneven wound edge

legal blindness. Visual acuity of 20/200 or less in the best corrected eye or peripheral visual of 20 degrees or less in the best corrected eye

lens. A transparent mass of tissue in the configuration of a biconvex lens enclosed within a rather tough capsule. It is supported by fine fibers (zonules) extending from the ciliary body, and its anterior surface rests on the posterior surface of the iris

light flashes. Reaction of the retina to stimulation by vitreous contraction tugging on vitreoretinal adhesions

light perception. A visual designation indicating that the best the patient can see is the appreciation of light

low-vision equipment. Magnification devices intended to assist people with vision not improvable to respectable levels by normal spectacle prescription

macular degeneration. A degenerative disease eventually resulting in the macula being destroyed—the result is loss of central vision

meibomian glands. Modified sebaceous glands that are embedded in the tarsus and exit at the lid margins. Their purpose is to produce an oily secretion to prevent tears from overflowing the lids

meibomitis. An infection of the meibomian gland. Ducts are not occluded and cyst does not form, as in chalazion

monocular vision. Seeing with one eye

mydriatic test. A test for narrow-angle glaucoma. The pupil is dilated (one eye at a time) with a short-acting mydriatic eyedrop. The elevation of intra-ocular pressure indicates possible narrow-angle glaucoma. Eyes are con-stricted at the end of the test

myopia. A condition in which the relaxed lens of the eye will focus parallel light rays (light rays from a distant object) in front of the retina so that they are then out of focus when they strike the retina

nevus. A nonelevated clump of pigment tissue, a mole. Nevi of the choroid must be differentiated from malignant melanoma

ocular dexter (O. D.). Right eye

ocular sinister (O. S.). Left eye

ocular uterque (O. U.). Both eyes

open-angle (chronic simple) glaucoma. A condition in which the intraocular pressure is elevated in the presence of an essentially normally appearing anterior chamber angle

optic neuritis. Inflammation of the optic nerve

orthoptics. Treatment by instruments involving exercises to help train the patient to use the eyes together

papilloma. An epithelial tumor, usually showing ridges or finger-like processes

perimetry. Technique of testing the peripheral retina or field of vision

peripheral fields. Test of the field of vision extending from fixation to the extreme periphery. Test is performed by plotting the patient's ability to see small targets on an arc 330 cm from the patient's eye

phacoemulsification. A surgical procedure for removal of cataracts. The lens is liquified by ultrasound waves and suctioned from the anterior chamber

phoria. A deviation of the eyes from the straight-ahead position when no stimulus to binocular vision is present

photocoagulation. The technique of causing a chorioretinal burn by using a concentrated light source focused through the pupil

plus-10 glasses. Plus-10 diopter glasses given to cataract patients in the early postoperative period as an approximation to the final glass requirement

primary congenital glaucoma. Glaucoma caused by incomplete embryologic development of the anterior chamber angle, resulting in reduction of aqueous outflow

prism. A transparent piece of glass or plastic in the form of a prism. It is used to measure the degree of crossed eyes and functions on the basis of its ability to change the direction of incoming light waves

prosthesis. A false eye

pterygium. A triangular fold of tissue that grows from the conjunctiva onto the cornea in the interpalpebral fissure usually on the medial side

ptosis. A condition in which the upper lid becomes partly or completely paralyzed so that it drops over the cornea

refraction. Technique of neutralizing abnormal focusing power of the eye

retina. A thin tissue composed primarily of nerve cells and their processes whose function is to convert light rays into nerve impulses. The retina lines the inside back wall of the eye and is closely adherent to the choroid. The retina is to the eye what film is to a camera

retinoblastoma. A malignant retinal tumor seen almost exclusively in infants

retinopathy. A rather loosely applied word indicating any type of retinal abnormality

retinoschisis. A condition in which the retina splits into two layers forming an intraretinal cyst

retrolental fibroplasia. A condition seen almost exclusively in premature infants who require supplemental oxygen. It results in preretinal fibrosis leading to distortion of the retina and, in extreme cases, total retinal detachment and blindness

sclera. The outer white fibrous coat of the eye. It forms the entire outer shell, except anteriorly where it blends in with the cornea

scleral depressor. An instrument used to indent the sclera. It is used in conjunction with ophthalmoscopy to examine the most anterior portion of the retina

slit-lamp biomicroscope. An instrument combining a microscope and a light source, used to examine the anterior segment of the eye. The light source may be narrowed so that it forms a slit of light—thus the name slit lamp

strabismus. A pathologic condition in which only one eye is directed at the intended object of regard

Sturge-Weber syndrome. A syndrome comprised of hemangioma of the face and of the pia mater. The size of the hemangioma may be extremely variable. Commonly, the hemangioma is called a port-wine stain. It is of interest to ophthalmology since the incidence of glaucoma in an eye surrounded by a facial hemangioma is rather high, and there is often an associated choroidal hemangioma

subconjunctival hemorrhage. A hemorrhage occurring under the bulbar conjunctiva. It stands out as a red blotch on the white sclera

synechiae. Adhesions between the iris and an adjacent structure

tarsal plate. Thin plates of dense fibrous tissue in the upper and lower lids that give shape and firmness to the lid

tonography. A technique used to study the outflow of aqueous from the anterior chamber

tonometer. An instrument used to measure intraocular pressure. Measurement is dependent on the indentation of the globe and a measurement of the force necessary to achieve indentation

toxocara canis. A parasitic infestation that may involve the eye. The ova are ingested, usually in dirt from areas where young dogs reside. The parasite then hatches and travels by blood vessel to the eye, where it causes an intense inflammatory response

toxoplasmosis. An intracellular parasitic disease that may involve the retina and cause a heavily pigmented chorioretinal scar with tendencies for reactivation

trailing. A technique taught to the blind, to allow them to examine their immediate surroundings by unostentatiously moving their fingers over the object at hand

tropia. A deviation of the eyes from normal position, a strabismus

ultrasonography. A technique using ultrasound waves to map the gross parameters of the globe. It is particularly useful in eyes with opaque corneas or cataracts

visual acuity. A measurement of visual discrimination. A standard means of measurement is the Snellen chart

vitreous body. Clear gel-like substance that fills the posterior portion of the eyeball

water drinking test. A provocative test for glaucoma. The test is predicated on the fact that drinking a large amount of water in a short amount of time (1 liter within 5 minutes) will cause a rapid increase in the aqueous production. If the outflow mechanism is compromised, the intraocular pressure will increase

zonules. The fibers that support the lens. They extend from the ciliary body to the equatorial region of the lens

INDEX

Abnormality, 11–15, 48–49, 103
Abrasion, 36, 44, 49–51
✳ Accommodation, 103, 245
Acid therapy, 18
Adhesions. *See* Synechiae
Age and aging process
  and cataracts, 119
  degenerative factor of, 38, 45, 164, 167,
    174, 266
  and retinal holes, 164, 200
Allergy, reaction to, 27, 37, 39, 154
Alpha-chymotrypsin, 122
Amblyopia, 108
Amblyoscope, 108–110
American Foundation for the Blind, 183
Anectine, 81
Anesthesia, general and topical, 16, 19,
  50–51, 113–115, 121–122
Angiography, use of, 93, 154, 157, 165,
  178–179, 192–195
Angle-closure glaucoma, 75, 83
Animals, spread of disease by, 163–164
Anterior chamber, 54, 65–88, 95–97
Antibiotic therapy, 8–13, 21–22, 27–30,
  38, 45, 49–52
Antiviral therapy, 42–43
Aphakia, 76, 80, 145, 211
Aqueous fluid
  outflow of, 71–73, 76, 84–87
  production of, 66
Arcuate scotoma, 71
Argyll Robertson pupil, 95
Arteriogram, 154
Artery, diseases of, 174–175
Arthritis, rheumatoid, 37, 90
Artificial eyeball. *See* Prosthesis
Assessment, techniques of, 248–251
Astigmatism, 154, 264–266
Atrophy, progression of, 75, 161, 170
Atropine, 66, 82, 87, 91, 114, 143, 208–
  209

Bacteria, involvement of, 39–40, 43–44,
  162–164
Biconvex glass lens, 117

Biomicroscope, 10, 34, 39, 120
Biopsy, 17, 19, 29
Bjerrum's scotoma, 71–72, 75
Black eye. *See* Ecchymosis
Black racial group, and sickle cell disease,
  192
Blepharitis, 9–10, 46
Blepharochalasis, 17
Blepharoconjunctivitis, 46
Blind spots, 71, 172
Blindness
  born in state of, 223
  cane usefulness for, 230
  fear of, 223
  legal status of, 143, 246
  night, 169
  partial low vision, 236–239
  and sensory loss, 223
  snow, 50
  training for, 108–110
Blockers, parasympathetic, 65–66
Blood, studies of, 90, 208
Blurred vision, 125–126, 202, 232
Bowman's membrane, 47, 50
Bruch's membrane, 151, 164–165
Burns
  acid, 52
  alkali, 52, 54, 284
  caustic, 39
  chemical, 23–24, 52, 284
  flash, 50
  solar, 50, 168
  sunlamp, 50
  thermal, 21–23, 39

Calcium, deposits of, 47
Canaliculus, 20–21
Cancer cells, 18–19, 29, 53. *See also*
  Tumor, malignant and nonmalignant
Carbachol, 76
Cataract, 164, 196, 211, 263
  age effect on, 119
  congenital, 119, 131–132
  and diabetes, 119
  hospital procedures, 125–127

DATE DUE			
DEC 2 8 1981			
APR 2 5 1982			
MAY 2 0 1983			
NOV 1 1 1990			
MAY 2 8 1993			
MAY 3 1 1993			
GAYLORD			PRINTED IN U.S.A.